GLASS IONOMER DENTAL CEMENT
— The Materials and Their Clinical Use —

Edited by:
Shigeru Katsuyama
Tatsuya Ishikawa
Benji Fujii

Ishiyaku EuroAmerica, Inc. Publishers
St. Louis • Tokyo

Editor, English Edition: Brian W. Cochran, M.F.A.
Advisor to the Editor: Arthur S. Wieselthier, Ph.D., D.M.D.

Ishiyaku EuroAmerica, Inc.
716 Hanley Industrial Court, St. Louis, Missouri 63144, U.S.A.
1-43-9, TS Bldg., #601, Komagome, Toshima-ku, Tokyo 170, JAPAN

Library of Congress Catalogue Card Number 92-53223

Shigeru Katsuyama, D.D.S., D.D.Sc.
Tatsuya Ishikawa, D.D.S., Ph.D., B.E.
Benji Fujii, D.D.S., D.Med.Sc.

English Traslation by Dawn E. Diehnelt, D.D.S.

GLASS IONOMER DENTAL CEMENT
— The Materials and Their Clinical Use —

ISBN 0-912791-94-2

Typesetting: Jennifer R. Little, M.A.
Printed in Japan

Contents

FOREWARD

An increasing interest in the use of glass ionomer cement is attributable to a number of factors. First, the cement has been improved in color, translucency, strength, and resistance to saliva. Second, clinical techniques have been developed that exploit the properties of the material to the maximum benefit of the patient. Finally, the glass ionomer/composite laminate restoration is gaining popularity and could extend the use of composite resins in clinical practice.

New concepts for treating both fissure and approximal caries take advantage of the adhesive properties of glass ionomer cement and its ability to leach fluoride. The glass ionomer/composite resin laminate may be the key to future developments in which the dentin is replaced with an adhesive, anticariogenic, and biologically compatible cement and the enamel with a translucent, abrasion-resistant composite material. The dentist may then be able to create a true replica of tooth structure which can survive long periods in a hostile environment.

Glass ionomer cement is the only restorative material that will form strong bonds to enamel and dentin in a moist environment. It is a material capable of further development, through metal-reinforced systems, higher molecular weight polyacids, and improved glasses, all of which may lead to the development of materials that could replace amalgam alloys.

The continuing efforts by GC Corp. to extend the opportunities for educating dentists in the latest technology in glass ionomer cement is greatly appreciated, and it is my great pleasure to write the foreward to this instructional book.

During the last 20 years, I have been privileged to work on the development of glass ionomer cement with Dr. Alan Wilson, my co-author in writing an earlier book on glass ionomer cement. For those wishing to increase their knowledge of the science and art of glass ionomer technology, this new book — published by Ishiyaku EuroAmerica — will complement the instructional literature published by GC Corp.

The future for the treatment of early caries lies within the glass ionomer field, and I predict that, with the use of fiber optic lighting, magnification, and micro-cutting of teeth, a new generation of children will grow up with their enamel preserved and with less fear of dental treatment. The future dental student should be taught these new techniques, and we must change our approach from macro- to micro-cutting of teeth so that these new adhesive materials can be used to their maximum advantage.

John W. McLean

INTRODUCTION

Glass ionomer cement was developed as a dental cement by A.D. Wilson and B.E. Kent, but the foundation for the birth of this new cement was laid in a long period of research on silicate cement. Ionomers are the product of inducing metal ionic bonding into an ethylene copolymer containing a carboxyl radical, and it can generally be said that glass ionomer cement is the product of silicate glass of alkaline earth metals reacting with an aqueous solution of acrylic acid. They are formally called alumino-silicate-polyacrylate cement, abbreviated as ASPA cement.

The powder is a glass of mostly alumina or silica acid. To make the glass, SiO_2, Al_2O_3, CaF_2, Na_3AlF_6, AlF_3, and $AlPO_4$ are melted at 1100-1300°C, cooled rapidly, and then made into a fine powder. The first liquid used for glass ionomer cement was an aqueous solution of polyacrylic acid, but now an aqueous solution of less than 50% copolymer of polyacrylic acid with either itaconic or maleic acid and approximately 5% tartaric acid added is used.

This cement was first produced by DeTrey Co. (Switzerland) and marketed by Amalgamated Dental Co. (England), Caulk Co. (U.S.), and others, and in the late 1970's, it came into clinical use in Europe and America. In Japan, the GC Corporation developed *Fuji Ionomer Cement* on its own in 1977, and because of subsequent improvements, this cement has become an indispensable product in the clinic today. It is used not only as a luting agent, but has also received much attention as a restorative material, a pit and fissure sealant, a liner, and as a dentin substitute.

Although glass ionomer cement has for some time been known to cause little irritation of the dental pulp, and also to achieve adhesive bonding with tooth structure and base metals, the first products had problems with basic physical properties such as water sensitivity and solubility. Now, however, actual clinical use has shown that the cement exhibits considerable durability and dramatically decreases dentin hypersensitivity in the cervical region.

Furthermore, the cement can be used as a liner, and secondary caries are repressed when it is used as a luting agent for cast restorations or as a restorative material, and restorative procedures using the cement are relatively simple. For these reasons, glass ionomer cement is now used clinically for purposes other than those for which composite resin restorations are used.

The caries rate for primary teeth and young permanent teeth has been decreasing recently, but concurrently we are becoming an older society. As a result, the time frame within which teeth are attacked has been lengthened, and cases of caries or defective restorations in the cervical region and root surface are increasing. As stated above, glass ionomer cement must now be recognized as an indispensable material for clinical use, and as such, its suitability extends over an extremely broad range.

Consequently, extensive research is being conducted in this area, and rapid developments in the field of material science are occurring. The reality, however, is that glass ionomer cement still exhibits many unsolved problems even as a restorative material, and little has been written about the cement.

This book is written especially for the clinician, and contains work of experts in their respective fields who have written about not only the theoretical background for glass ionomers, but also about their actual clinical use, including specific techniques. Naturally, academic progress does not stop, and one can surmise that it will be necessary to revise this book in a few years. I would therefore like to solicit suggestions from our readers in order to make a more complete book in the future.

Shigeru Katsuyama
Editor-in-Chief

CHAPTER I

THE DEVELOPMENT OF GLASS IONOMER CEMENT

THE DEVELOPMENT OF GLASS IONOMER CEMENT

Benji Fujii
Department of Restorative Dentistry
Osaka Dental College

Early Development

Glass ionomer cement was developed by A.D. Wilson (Fig. 1-1), head researcher at the English Laboratory of the Government Chemist, and his colleague B.E. Kent. Glass ionomer cement was, from the very beginning, the center of enthusiastic research on dental cement, specifically research on improving the basic properties of silicate cement.

Wilson and Kent's Glass ionomer cement was found to maximize the positive qualities of the silicate cement while minimizing its negative properties. All at once, glass ionomer cement was spotlighted as a new material which could adhere to tooth structure. A patent was applied for in 1969, and the research results were published in the *British Dental Journal* (1972) under the title "A New Translucent Cement for Dentistry." Since then, new research results on glass ionomer cement have continually been published in this journal.

Actually, polycarboxylate cement was developed by D.C. Smith (1968)[A1] before glass ionomer cement, and it is not hard to imagine that the new carboxylate cement was an important force in giving rise to glass ionomer cement. The powder in glass ionomer cement is calcium aluminosilicate glass, and the liquid is the same as that in polycarboxylate cement, a copolymer formed by adding itaconic acid to polyacrylic acid. This liquid has subsequently been adjusted so as to maintain a constant viscosity, and furthermore, researchers have tried to make the cement set more sharply by adding a small amount of tartaric acid.

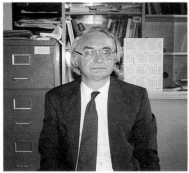

Fig. 1-1. Dr. Wilson (1979, Laboratory of the Government Chemist).

When glass ionomer cement was initially developed, the first letters of alumino-silicate glass, the powder, and polyacrylic acid, the liquid, were used to form the acronym "ASPA." The De Trey Company (Switzerland) manufactured this cement, and the Amalgamated Dental Company (England) and Caulk Company (U.S.A.) were the distributors. The product was first sold in Europe and the United States under its abbreviated name, *ASPA Cement*, as a restorative material (Fig. 1-2), with actual clinical use beginning in Europe around 1975, and in North America in around 1977.

In the meantime, the GC Corp. undertook development of a similar product on its own in Japan, and produced *Fuji Ionomer Type I* (Fig. 1-3) as a luting cement (1977).

Since then, these manufacturers have continued to develop the product, and the ESPE Company of Germany, the Shofu Company of Japan, and others have also begun to produce the cement. Many new products have emerged and are available today.

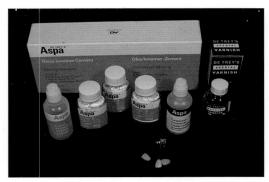

Fig. 1-2. *ASPA Cement* (De Trey Co.) and related products.

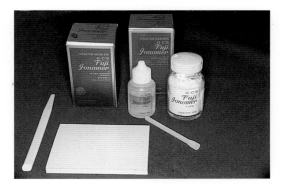

Fig. 1-3. *Fuji Ionomer Type I* (GC Corp.) and mixing instruments.

Improvements

Many improvements have been made since De Trey's *ASPA Cement* was first sold, and here I will briefly touch on the major points.

The Powder

The powder is basically calcium aluminosilicate glass, but the relative amounts of silica, alumina, and calcium fluoride may vary between different manufacturers. In water-hardening glass ionomer cement, the liquid component of the polyacrylic acid is included in the powder as a polymer.

Depending on the intended use of the cement, pigments, zinc oxide, radiopaque materials, and pure silver or a silver alloy (amalgam) may be added to the powder. Many different products are thus now available, some with tannin fluoride.

Changes in the Liquid

The early *ASPA Cement*, following Wilson's original formula, used a copolymer of polyacrylic and itaconic acids, but some producers today use maleic or other acids in place of the itaconic acid.

Water-hardening cement, in which the carboxylates such as polyacrylic acid are removed from the liquid, has now appeared, mostly from European manufacturers. The main advantage of water-hardened glass ionomer cement is that accurate measurement is facilitated because the viscosity of the liquid does not change.

As A Restorative Cement

As stated earlier, glass ionomer cement first appeared on the market as *ASPA Cement*, and thereafter, *Fuji Ionomer Type I* was marketed by the GC Corp., a Japanese firm. The competition between these two products continued for some time, and thus the two cements became the object of comparison. The De Trey Company then developed *Chemfil*, a water-hardening cement, as an improvement over its own *ASPA Cement*, and the ESPE Company entered the market with *Ketac-Fil* (in capsules) and *Chelon-Fil* (in bottles), both water-hardening polymaleic glass ionomer cements. The esthetics and ease of handling found in restorative glass ionomer cement began to show marked progress.

Fuji Ionomer Type II appeared on the market after the *Type I* luting cement, and gained a worldwide reputation for superior esthetics and ease of handling compared to the *ASPA Cement*, and thus this new cement contributed greatly to the widespread use of glass ionomer cement. The Shofu Company in Japan then entered the development race, and began marketing a plain glass ionomer cement as well as *Hy-Bond* glass ionomer cement, a cement with tannin fluoride added.

When the physical and mechanical properties of restorative glass ionomer cement are considered, it is clear that it should be used as a material for the Class 3 and Class 5 regions of anterior teeth (which demand esthetics) rather than in regions subject to strong occlusal forces.

Glass ionomer cement competes with composite resins, but is especially useful for cases of cervical abrasion (especially with hypersensitivity) and for root caries. The cement's adhesive strength to tooth structure is certainly not great, but the cement has superior retention, a tight marginal seal, and is safe for the pulp. Some people have even reported that the cement restorations do not fall out for a long time even in cavities with limited retention form. [19]

There is little discoloration, and staining of the margins seldom occurs. Glass ionomer cement also has the highly desirable clinical property of leading to an extremely low rate of secondary caries around restorations. Only after a great deal of time in the oral cavity, when the cement restoration may dissolve slightly, does a slight breakdown of the margins easily occur.

As a Luting Cement

Type I Fuji Ionomer was the first glass ionomer marketed as a luting agent, but at that time, fine powderization of the particles was difficult, so the film thickness of the cement was apt to be large. More than a few people doubted its clinical application as a luting cement.

Wilson et al,[11] realizing that there was a problem with glass ionomer as a luting agent, tried to improve the cement, and finally made a test product called *ASPA IV-A*. This was a major step toward the effective use of glass ionomer as a luting cement. Furthermore, Wilson and his colleagues stated at that time that the adhesion of glass ionomer luting cement to precious metals was unstable and that the problem should be solved by tin-plating the interior surface of precious metal castings.

Reisbeck[13] then compared the various clinical qualities of *Chembond*, the product produced by De Trey Company for *ASPA IV-A*, with other luting cements, and reported that glass ionomer cement was suitable as a luting cement.

After that, water-hardening *Ketac-Cem* (ESPE Co.) and *Aqua Cem* (De Trey Co.) were marketed, earning acclaim from clinicians because of improvements in handling and solubility which they represented.

The physical, chemical, and handling properties of glass ionomer luting cement have been greatly improved since the cement was first developed. In particular, the film thickness has become smaller. These improvements, coupled with the cement's compatibility with the pulp, has caused its reputation as a luting cement to take a large step up. Specifically, many practitioners now think that the cement is ideal for cases involving relatively large dental pulps when postoperative hypersensitivity is feared. However, because of its relatively short working time, it is unfit for cementing bridges with several abutments.

Dilts et al[D21] have studied the cement's adhesive strength with amalgam, composite resin, gold alloys and nickel-chromium alloys and found that there was a problem in particular with its adhesive strength to core materials. Kitano,[D32] however, reported that, if one is merely careful about protecting the glass ionomer after luting, it adheres with almost as much strength as to dentin, and if this is indeed the case, then there appears to be no need to worry.

As a Liner and Base

The superior properties which glass ionomer cement exhibits as a restorative material have been noted, but the truth is that its mechanical strength as a restorative material, especially tensile strength and resistance to plastic deformation, are low: when durability is a prime concern, the inferiority of glass ionomer cement to composite resins cannot be denied.

Nevertheless, I believe that if this material is used as a lining or base directly under restorative materials, it exhibits wonderful characteristics that simply are not found in other materials.

Actually, the cement's ideal properties

can only be realized when it is used as a material for linings or bases. Recently many new glass ionomer products have been put on the market for just such a purpose. If we learn to skillfully utilize these products, the likelihood of attaining an epoch-making advancement in the restoration of hard tissue diseases such as caries is great.

As a Liner

In 1977, McLean et al[K1] were the first to recommend lining composite resins with glass ionomer cement by filling the cement up to the dentoenamel junction and the placing composite resin over it.

Lining Cement marketed by the GC Corp. in 1983, was the first cement in the world developed specifically for lining composite resin restorations. Zinc oxide was added to the basic glass ionomer cement, and the degree of polymerization of the polyacrylic acid was lowered to decrease the viscosity of the liquid so that it could be placed on the cavity floor and spread as thinly as possible. This cement is semi-transparent, has a snap set, and is radiopaque. This product was welcomed by many clinicians, and has been used regularly in the U.S. and several other countries as a glass ionomer liner with good handling properties. It has been well received.

Spurred by this development, the ESPE Co. began to market *Ketac Bond*, and the Shofu Co., which had emphasized carboxylate cement, recently began to market *HY-Bond Liner*. These products allow a one-step lining process, a whole new concept which is quite different from the original zinc phosphate cement lining.

As a Base or Build-Up

Prior to the improvement of glass ionomer cement, the use of a dry mix of zinc phosphate cement as a base for restoring molars with amalgam or metal inlays had become common sense. The zinc phosphate cement was widely used by clinicians for many years, due to its advantages of ideal strength, good handling, and radiopacity.

However, zinc phosphate does not bond to dentin, so the seal was inferior, and there was also irritation of the pulp. A further disadvantage was that its use was limited to non-extensive cases only. To overcome that disadvantage, *Base Cement* was introduced by the Shofu Co. as the first glass ionomer cement in the world designed specifically for bases.

Color and radiopacity have been added to Shofu's high strength glass ionomer in this cement, available in three colors—white, red and dentin. The cement has an elasticity similar to that of dentin, it bonds to surrounding dentin, and the seal is tight. Furthermore, due to the cement's fluoride release, one can expect repression of secondary caries. This cement can be used as a base not only for metal inlays and amalgam restorations, but also for core buildups, and of course with composite resins.

At about the same time, the ESPE Co. developed *Glass Cermet Cement* with McLean. This product contains silver and aluminosilicate glass sintered together and ground into a powder,[M2] and has been marketed as *Ketac Silver* mainly in Europe and North America, where it has received good appraisals. This product is designed for the same objectives as *Base Cement*, and can also be used as a temporary restorative material for molars.

To achieve similar objectives, an American practitioner (J. J. Simmons) recommended a simpler method of mixing a relatively high proportion of amalgam powder (i.e., about the same quantity as the cement powder) with the cement powder, and then mixing this with cement liquid. This was called the "Miracle-Mixture" method,[M1] and the commercial product based on this idea is called *Miracle Mix* (GC Corp.). Many people routinely use this product in the U.S. Recently, the GC Corp. has developed *Dentin Cement* for the same purpose.

Use on Cervix and Roots

Cervical Cement has only recently been marketed by the GC Corp.: this cement has a lowered viscosity for the treatment of hyper-sensitive root areas.

As a Pit and Fissure Sealant

The potential of glass ionomer cement as a promising pit and fissure sealant has been suggested by McLean et al[L5] since the cement's early development, but it was not until 1986 that the GC Corp. marketed *Fuji Ionomer Type III Cement* as a product specifically for this use. According to Shimokobe et al, the cement's viscosity is low and its fluoride release is excellent. Durability in the oral cavity is not as great as that of the resin-type sealants, but one must also consider that more than just mechanically sealing the fissure, the cement's fluoride release creates resistance to caries in the enamel. In fact, the objective in using glass ionomer cement as a fissure sealant should be different than that in using resin sealants.

CHAPTER II

THE COMPOSITION AND SETTING REACTION OF GLASS IONOMER CEMENT

THE COMPOSITION AND SETTING REACTION OF GLASS IONOMER CEMENT

Hiroyasu Hosoda
Department of Restorative Dentistry
Tokyo Medical and Dental College

Glass Ionomer Cement

Powder

Similar to the powder of silicate cements, the powder of glass ionomer cement is finely ground ceramic glass, and is soluble in acid. The main components of the powder are silica (SiO) and alumina (Al_2O_3), and the following may be added to this mixture: calcium fluoride (CaF_2) as flux, cryolite (Na_3AlF_3), sodium fluoride (NaF), and/or aluminum phosphate ($AlPO_4$). These are fused at about 1100-1500° C (the temperature varies depending on the composition of the melting particles), and the paste-like glass is then rapidly cooled and ground into the powder used for glass ionomer cement.

The particle size found in the powder used for restorative materials or lining cement is rather large—with most particles being about 45 μm in diameter—but the particle size in the powder used for luting cement or pit and fissure sealant is less than 25 μm.

Table 2-1 shows the composition of glass ionomer cement powders. G200 is the formula of A.D. Wilson, the developer of glass ionomer cement,[B9,10,29] and should be referred to as the pioneer form of glass ionomer cement. The amount of CaF_2 has been decreased, and the Al_2O_3/SiO_2 ratio has been changed in modern day cement to improve esthetics and the degree of transparency, as can be seen in products A and B (Table 2-1).[A40]

In water-hardening cement, components which contribute to the setting reaction are mixed into the powder, and cement forma-

Table 2-1. Composition of glass ionomer cement powders.

| Component | Powder composition of several types of glass ionomer cement | | | |
	A	B	G200	water hardening cement
SiO_2	41.9	35.2	29.0	5 parts glass powder of various components 1 part copolymer high molecular acid 0.1 part tartaric acid
Al_2O_3	28.6	20.1	16.5	
CaF_2	15.7	20.1	34.3	
$F1F_3$	1.6	2.4	7.3	
$AlPO_4$	3.8	12.0	9.9	
NaF	9.3	3.6	3.0	

tion is initiated by mixing the powder with water.[I6]

Liquid

The liquid used to make the cement is a solution of high molecular electrolytes.

Table 2-2 shows the composition of the liquid of glass ionomer cement.[B11,I6] Liquid A was used in the test of *ASPA* (aluminosilicate polyacrylate) *Type 1*. This 50% aqueous solution of polyacrylic acid (molecular weight 2,300) was tried in the pioneer types of glass ionomer cement. However, when the G200 glass powder was mixed with this liquid, two problems were encountered.

The setting speed was long, and the liquid turned into a gel over time and became unusable. By adding tartaric acid to the high molecular electrolytic solution (polyacrylic acid solution) as a chelating agent, the setting speed was improved. However, there remained the problem of preserving the

16

cement liquid (Table 2-2, Liquid B), as it would become a gel in 20 to 30 weeks, depending on the product. The first treatment used to prevent gelation was the methylation of a portion of the carboxyl radical, with the hydrogen bonding then suppressing gelation (Table 2-2, Liquid C). However, since the cement using Liquid C was weaker than that using either Liquid A or B, a new way of suppressing gelation had to be devised.

The answer was to manufacture a new liquid using a copolymer of acrylic and itaconic acids (molecular weight 10,400; see Fig. 2-1). This copolymer has less regularity than polyacrylic acid, and condensation by hydrogen bonding is hindered, so this copolymer is stable over a long period of time and does not become a gel (Table 2-2, Liquid D). Copolymers of acrylic and maleic acids are also similarly stable and do not gel. The formula of each company for the liquids used today are confidential and cannot be stated precisely, but in general, copolymers such as can be seen in Figure 2-1 (or with a few added adornments) are used.

Additionally, when the high molecular electrolytes are freeze-dried and mixed into

Table 2-2. Composition of glass ionomer liquid.

mixed with	code composition of the cement liquids	liquid composition
acid	A	aqueous solution of 50% polyacrylic acid
	B	aqueous solution of 47.5% polyacrylic acid, 5% tartaric acid
	C	aqueous solution of 47.5% polyacrylic acid, 5% tartaric acid, 5% methanol
	D	aqueous solution of 47.5% copolymer of acrylic/itaconic acid (2:1), 5% tartaric acid
	E	aqueous solution of 47.5% copolymer of acrylic/maleic acid, 5% tartaric acid
water	F	aqueous solution of 10% tartaric acid
	G	pure water

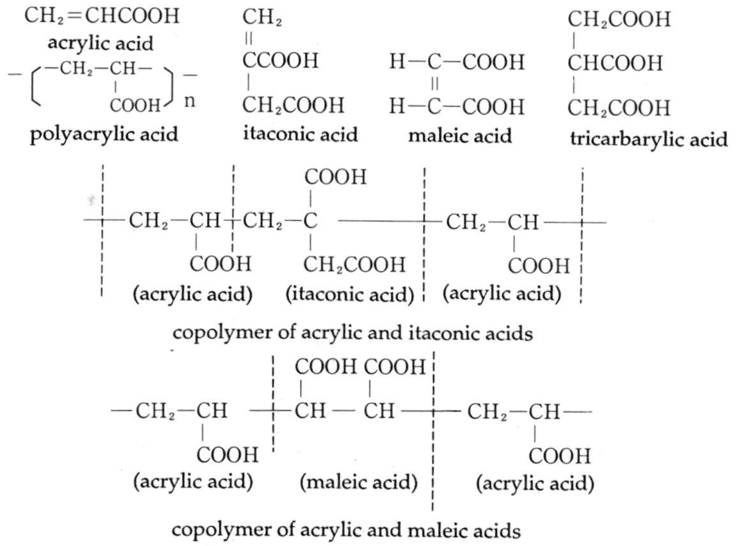

Fig. 2-1. Major acids used in glass ionomer cement.

the powder as particles, they are, like F and G in Table 2-2, then mixed with either water or an aqueous solution of tartaric acid to form the cement paste.

The Setting Reaction

The setting reaction of glass ionomer cement is basically an acid-base reaction, but the process is quite complicated, and moreover, not completely understood. However, a plausible explanation can be arrived at by mixing in a little hypothesis. Understanding the principles involved in the setting reaction of this cement is extremely important for clinicians using it in the oral cavity. The reaction starts as soon as the liquid contacts the surface of the powder.

Initial Reaction

When the powder and liquid are mixed together, they form a paste, and the powder, being basic, readily reacts with the high-molecular acids (polyalkenoic acids such as polyacrylic acid) which make up the liquid. The first stage of the reaction is the ionization of the carboxyl radical (COOH) to COO⁻ (carboxylate ion) and H⁺, and the H⁺ ion (positive) acts first on the surface of the glass particles (Table 2-2, b).

If the powder particles were composed only of silica (SiO_2), the powder would not be attacked by the acid. But when there is aluminosilicate which includes calcium (calcium aluminosilicate), like there is in the powder of cement made with alumina (Al_2O_3), the AlO_4 and SiO_4 jointly share the O's around them, and some of the silicon in the silicic acid is replaced by aluminum. The portion which will become the basic glass (AlO_4) becomes negatively charged, and is then readily attacked and taken away by the acid. The aluminosilicate usually has a chain-like, stratified, rope-like structure, and the positive ions lie in the spaces (Fig. 2-3, a).

In such a manner, the attack by the H⁺ ion begins, and in the very early stages of the reaction, the ions adorning the glass (Ca^{2+}, Na^+) are released into the liquid.

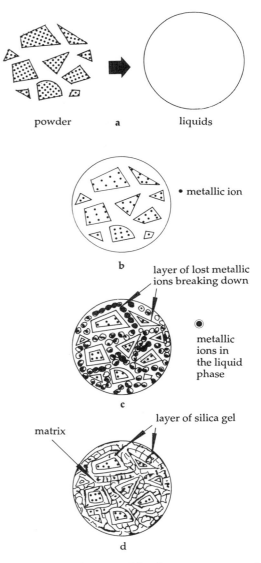

Fig. 2-2. Coagulation and hardening processes of glass ionomer cement.

a. Mixing glass powder and cement liquid.

b. The COOH radical attached to the polyacrylic acid chain ionizes to COO⁻ and H⁺, and the H⁺ (the positive ion) attacks the glass surfaces.

c. Ca⁺ and Al³⁺ are released into the liquid phase by the H⁺ attack on the glass surface, and it becomes a layer of lost metallic ions (*arrow*), in time forming a layer of silica gel. The released ions start the gelation.

d. As the reaction proceeds, silica gel is formed by the condensation reaction surrounding the glass, and insoluble polyacrylate precipitates in the matrix, and as it hardens, hydration proceeds and a highly hydrated gel is formed.

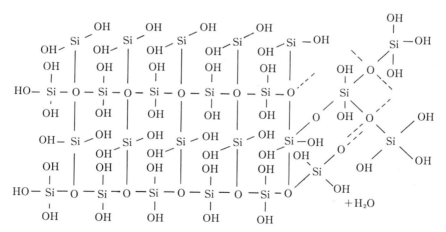

Fig. 2-3. Formation of silica gel.
  a. Calcium aluminosilicate.
  b. Breakdown of aluminosilicate and release
     of the Al^{3+} by the H^+ ion.
  c. Formation of silica gel.

The H+ ion then penetrates again into the rather disorganized structure, and the Al³⁺ ion is dissolved away. When this happens, the aluminosilicate glass is broken down into silicic acid (H_4SiO_4; see Fig. 2-3, b). This silicic acid slowly causes a condensation reaction by means of its OH radical, and becomes a porous silica gel having a rope-like structure (Fig. 2-3, c), and the unreacted glass particles (core) become surrounded (Fig. 2-2, c) with gel.

In effect, the outer surface of the glass powder is attacked by acid, and at first the Ca²⁺ ions and a small number of Na⁺ ions are released and move into the liquid. In the next step, the Al³⁺ ions are released, but rather than being individual ions in and of themselves, it is thought that they migrate as AlF^{2+} and AlF^{2+}.[B2] Through this process, the surface layer of the glass powder becomes a layer in which almost all metallic ions are lost, and the region becomes silica gel.

Gel Formation

The concentration of ions in the cement liquid gradually becomes greater, and along with this, the pH rises. This rise in pH indicates that the polyacrylic acid reacts with metallic ions with a charge of more than two and is slowly transformed into a cross-linked metallic salt, i.e., polyacrylate. Naturally, viscosity increases.

When the polyacrylic metallic salt begins to precipitate in the liquid, gelation starts, and the reaction proceeds further and the cement hardens. Even after the initial stages of condensation, the precipitation of salts proceeds until all of the metallic ion becomes insoluble (Fig. 2-2, c). The initial condensation is from calcium polyacrylate, and later, large quantities of aluminum polyacrylate are slowly formed, hardening the cement.

One must be careful at this point because the cement is readily affected by water immediately after the initial condensation. There are fluoride and metallic ions (especially Al⁺ ions) in the cement at this initial

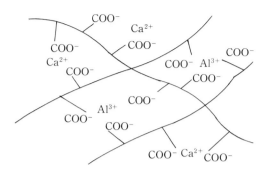

Fig. 2-4. Diagram of a high molecular electrolyte (such as polyacrylic acid) and the crosslink bonding with Ca²⁺ and Al³⁺. (It is difficult to think of Al³⁺ bonding with 3 chains.)

stage which have not yet reacted with polyacrylic acid, as well as ions which are in the process of reacting with polyacrylic acid, and furthermore there is newly formed calcium polyacrylate, and all of these are in a soluble state. Once there is contact with water, the above are liquidated and the formation of a strong matrix is prevented. As a result, the cement weakens and whitens. The Na⁺ ion becomes only sodium polyacrylate, a viscous substance, and does not become a gel.

Metallic Salt Formation

The main metallic ions released into the cement liquid are the +2 charged Ca²⁺ and the 3+ charged Al³⁺. These crosslink with two or three COO⁻ ions of the chain of polyacrylic acid, and it is thought that this becomes a gel (Fig. 2-4). This gel is hydrated, and its strength increases as the hydrated gel structure progresses.

In general, when metallic ions are dissolved in water, they become an alcohol with a water molecule, becoming a complex ion with six waters ($M(OH_2)_6)^{2+}$). This complex ion with a 2+ charge can react with the negative ion COO⁻ of the high molecular electrolytes,[B7] so rather than thinking that the Ca²⁺ ion is the only main ion crosslink-

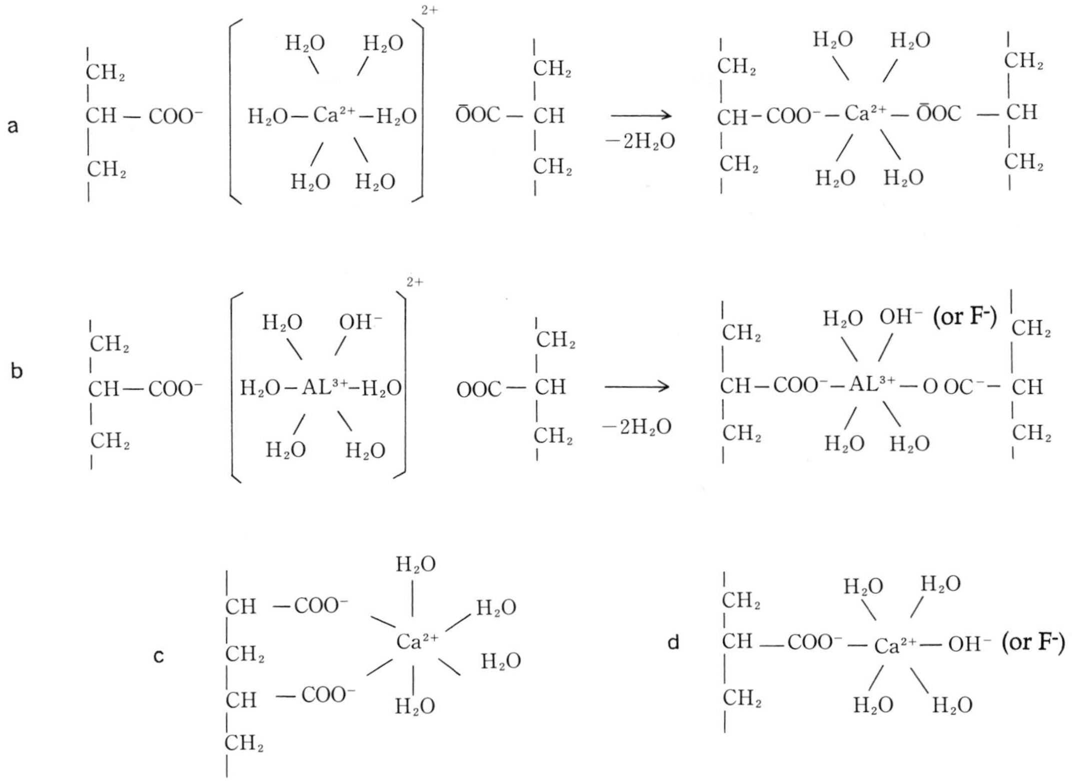

Fig. 2-5. Hypothesized formation of polyacrylate with Ca or Al and the molecular structure.

ing, there are those that conjecture that it reacts in the form of $(Ca(OH_2)_6)^{2+}$. This makes it easier to explain the increase of water bonding and the hydration reaction (Fig. 2-5, a).

Three COO⁻ (carboxylate ions) are necessary for the 3+ charged Al^{3+} to react completely, but as it is difficult to think of this as a rigid structure, one can reasonably believe that it, similar to Ca^{2+}, reacts with two COO⁻.[B9] That is, both the Al and Ca have a configuration number of six, so the freed Al^{3+} ion is hydrated in the liquid and forms $(Al(OH_2)_6)^{3+}$, an alcohol ion. This ion is a weak base, and it is hydrolyzed in the water. $(Al(O_2H)_6)^{3+} + H_2O \rightleftarrows H_30^+ + (Al(OH_2)_5OH)^{2+}$

This 2+ charged complex ion $(Al(OH_2)_5OH)^{2+}$ reacts like the complex ion of Ca^{2+} and crosslinks with two COO⁻. This is a satisfactory way of explaining how it is thought that aluminum polyacrylate is formed. The OH⁻ ion and the F⁻ ion are the same size, so these sections are easily interchanged.

Figure 2-5c shows another bonding form of Ca^{2+}.[B7] The complete reaction is difficult to explain clearly because it involves a mixture of complex ions, with F⁻ ion and tartaric acid in addition to the above reaction process.

Setting

Polyacrylate is an insoluble salt and hardens (Fig. 2-2, d). The precipitation of polyacrylic salts, especially aluminum salts, and the setting that follows, continues for over 24 hours, as transparency is gradually manifested. The setting process continues thereafter, but only at a minute pace, for

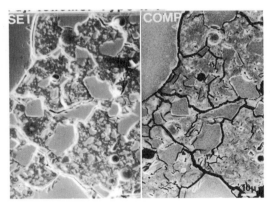

Fig. 2-6. Scanning electron micrograph of hardened *Fuji Ionomer Cement Type II-F*. SEI: secondary electronic image, COMP: composite image.

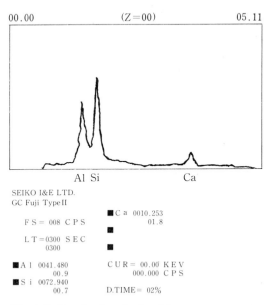

00.00   (Z＝00)   05.11

Al Si   Ca

SEIKO I&E LTD.
GC Fuji Type II

     F S ＝ 008 C P S

     L T ＝0300 S E C
       0300

■ C a   0010.253
       01.8
■

■

■ A l   0041.480
     00.9
■ S i   0072.940
     00.7

C U R ＝ 00.00 K E V
    000.000 C P S

D.TIME＝ 02%

Fig. 2-7. Graph of analysis of the same cement.

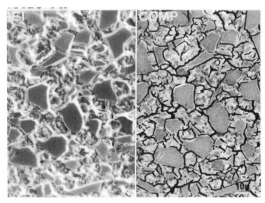

Fig. 2-8. Scanning electron micrograph of hardened *Ketac-Fil Cement*. SEI: secondary electronic image, COMP: composite image.

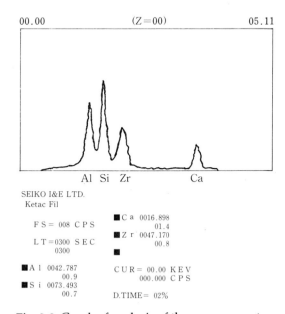

00.00   (Z＝00)   05.11

Al Si Zr   Ca

SEIKO I&E LTD.
Ketac Fil

     F S ＝ 008 C P S

     L T ＝0300 S E C
       0300

■ C a   0016.898
       01.4
■ Z r   0047.170
       00.8
■

■ A l   0042.787
     00.9
■ S i   0073.493
     00.7

C U R ＝ 00.00 K E V
    000.000 C P S

D.TIME＝ 02%

Fig. 2-9. Graph of analysis of the same cement.

about a year. Over the first few days, the transparency of the cement continually increases, and the cement is not susceptible to drying; it exhibits sufficient strength and hardness. The increase in strength and hardness is due to the increasing content of aluminum polyacrylate with adequate crosslinking, and also because these metallic salts hydrate, and the gel structure of hydrated elements expands much more.

Water in the cement liquid plays an important role in the formation of a hydrated gel, as can be seen in the formation of the metallic polyacrylates (Fig. 2-5), so water cannot be limiting factor in the formation of the silica gel.

Figures 2-6 through 2-9 show scanning electron micrographs of hardened cement, and graphs analyzing the cement composition. Cracks appeared in the cement due to the drying which was needed to make the micrograph. A composite image is shown, and as can be seen in the secondary electron image, cracks are apparent between the silica gel structure around the powder particles and the matrix (substrate). One can question whether the substrate, (i.e., the hydrolyzed polyacrylate) withstood drying and whether a strong bond formed. Additionally, Zr was detected along with Al, Si, and Ca in the analysis of *Ketac-Fil* (German ESPE Co.).

Fluoride and Tartaric Acid in the Setting Reaction

Fluoride

The cement powder of the first publicly available glass ionomer contained a large quantity of fluoride (G200, Table 2-1). The addition of fluoride improved handling properties, and these properties could easily be altered by changing the amount of fluoride added. The presence of fluoride, especially the F^- ion, contributes a lot to the formation of complex bodies, with the metallic ions released into the liquid. It becomes CaF^+ and AlF^{2+}, and delays the bonding of the positive ions with either polyacrylic acid (a high molecular acid) to

form polyacrylate (Ca^{2+}, Al^{3+}), or with the COO^- in the copolymer chains. The process of gelation is slowed for these reasons, and working time can thus be lengthened. The formation of complex bodies quickens the release of the hydrogen ion ($H+$), lowering the pH of the paste, and the gelation, which depends on the pH, is also slowed.

Tartaric Acid

The fact that the handling characteristics of glass ionomer cement is improved by the formation of complex bodies by the fluoride provided a clue for Wilson et al,[B13] and they set out to find a chelating agent.

It was found that optically active L-tartaric acid with two asymmetric carbon molecules and two COOH radicals was particularly effective as such an agent. Tartaric acid can form a cement because it has two COOH radicals, but the resulting cement is unstable in water.

The action of tartaric acid on glass ionomer cement is unclear, but when tartaric acid is mixed in, the very early stages of the reaction occur between tartaric acid and the surface of the powder, since it is a stronger acid than polyacrylic acid. That is, the formation of complex bodies with complex bonding to the positive ions in solution or salts of tartaric salt (calcium tartrate) occurs first because of the attack by the acid.

The formation of these complex bodies plays the same role as that stated for the fluoride ion. Consequently, handling properties improve, and the fluoride content in the glass can be decreased. This is then related to improvements in the translucency of the hardened cement.

As the Ca^{2+} released from the glass surface reacts selectively with the tartaric acid, calcium tartrate is formed, and it is thought that this also contributes to the initial condensation.[B9]

It is believed that the compound of the metallic ions and the complex bodies have a structure like that shown in Figure 2-10,[B9] and it appears as though the metallic ions have a role as a temporary helping hand. As

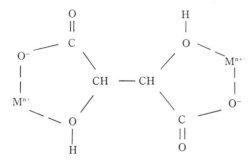

Fig. 2-10. Complex body of metallic ions and tartaric acid.

the condensation reaction progresses, the ions are released and soon react with the polyacrylic acid. The significance of adding tartaric acid to the glass ionomer cement system is great, and the following special characteristics are exhibited as a result.[B9,13]

1. The mixing of the cement paste is improved, and an appropriate working time can be obtained.

2. Setting is sharp. That is, after a certain elapsed time, the cement hardens very quickly.

3. The strength of the cement is increased.

4. As stated above, since the fluoride content can be decreased, transparency and esthetics can be improved.

CHAPTER III

PROPERTIES
AND
CHARACTERISTICS

PROPERTIES AND CHARACTERISTICS
Section 1: Physical and Mechanical Properties

Hideo Onose
Department of Preventive Dentistry, Restorative Section
Nihon University Dental School

Glass ionomer cement is generally used as a luting cement, lining, or restorative material, and products with different properties have been developed for each use.

Luting Glass Ionomers

The properties of commercial products in their set and unset states are shown in Table 3-1. The following are the required properties for luting cement.

1. Appropriate working time and good handling properties

These are important factors related to how easy the cement is to use in the clinic. It is desirable for the powder and liquid of the cement, when mixed, to reach a paste-like consistency easily, and further, the cement should not set until the luting procedures are completed. With these requirements, one sees that zinc phosphate, the typical luting cement used in the past, has lengthy instructions because different physical properties occur depending on how the cement is mixed. However, with glass ionomer cement, there are few rules for mixing; the prescribed amount of powder and liquid can be mixed all at once, and it can even be done mechanically.

A standard viscosity for cement used in luting restorations has been established, but when this standard is applied to glass ionomer cement with the standard powder-

Table 3-1. Properties of luting glass ionomers.

Data for Japanese products provided by manufacturer.
Data for other products from research reports.

	Fuji I	HY-Bond C	Ketac-Cem	zinc phosphate	ISO 77489 Type I
Manufacturer	GC	Shofu	ESPE		
Major usage	luting	luting	luting	luting	luting
Standard powder:liquid ratio	1.8/1.0	1.5/1.0	3.4/1.0		
Initial set	5'30"	5'15"	7'00"	7'00"	~7'30"
Compressive greater than strength (kg/cm^2)	1800	2006	1200	1100	663(65MPa)
Diametral tensile strength (kg/cm^2)	89	97	77	47	
Film thickness (μm)	18	22	22	18	less than 25
Solubility less than 1.0	0.08	0.30	0.40	0.06	(1 day, %)
Surface hardness (Hv, after 1 day)	48				
Coefficient of thermal expansion	10.7x10^{-6}				
Radiopacity	+	−	−	+	−
Adhesive strength (kg/cm^2) enamel dentin	51 37		50		

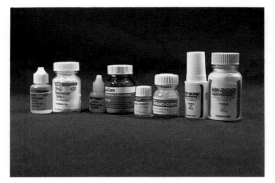

Fig. 3-1. Luting glass ionomer cement.

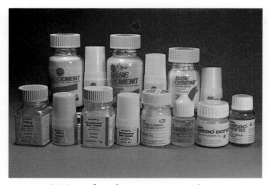

Fig. 3-2. Lining glass ionomer cement.

to-liquid ratio, the viscosity is rather high. Because the viscosity of the glass ionomer liquid is higher than that of zinc phosphate, glass ionomer cement has been criticized as being difficult to mix. Recently, however, easy-to-mix products have been marketed in response to these criticisms; the composition of the liquid has been changed, and the powderization of the powder particles has been improved. However, since the setting time of this luting cement is relatively short (5 minutes and 30 seconds), the feeling that the procedure is rushed persists.

2. Good physical properties

A large part of maintaining restorations in cavity preparations depends on the interlocking forces created as a result of the cement being forced into the fine spaces between the restoration and the cavity walls. This principle holds true even for glass ionomer cement, which bonds chemically to tooth structure and some metals. Compressive strength is a representative physical property related to these interlocking forces. Glass ionomer cement has a relatively high compressive strength, with values of any of the products surpassing established standards, so the interlocking forces are also high.

3. Thin film thickness

The film thickness of luting cement is an important factor in seating restorations to their proper position on the prepared tooth. Recently, because of advancements in pro-

ducing restorations which fit accurately onto the preparation, the property of film thickness has become connected with handling properties, contributing to the evaluation of how easy the cement is to use.

Glass ionomer cement was first criticized because of its thick film thickness, but recent products have about the same values as zinc phosphate.

4. Other required properties

Other required properties of luting cement are: low solubility in the fluids of the oral cavity; little injury to the pulp and periodontal tissues; good wetting of the restoration and tooth structure; and if possible, adhesion. These three topics will be explained in detail in the following sections, because glass ionomer cement has special characteristics which should be dealt with in detail. In any case, these three are important requirements of any luting cement.

Liner & Base Glass Ionomers

The properties of representative commercial products in their set and unset states are shown in Table 3-2.

The following are the required properties for lining cement (Fig. 3-2).

1. Good physical properties

The extent to which various physical properties should be demonstrated in lining materials is debatable, but lining materials can be thought of as substitutes for lost dentin. In other words, the physical proper-

Table 3-2. Properties of lining glass ionomers.

	Lining	Dentin	Base (Pink)	Base (Dentin)	Base (White)	Ketac-Bond	Dentin	Standard Type II
Manufacturer	GC	GC	Shofu	Shofu	Shofu	ESPE		
Major usage	Lining	Lining	Lining	Lining	Lining	Lining		
Standard powder:liquid ratio	1.2/1.0	2.2/1.0	2.4/1.0	2.6/1.0	2.6/1.0	3.4/1.0		
Initial set	4'00"	3'45"	4'00"	4'30"	4'30"			~5'00"
Compressive strength (kg/cm^2)	750	1880	2300	2350	2350	1500	2800	>1275(125MPa)
Diametral tensile strength (kg/cm^2)			91		98			
Solubility (1 day, %)	0.50	0.05	0.33	0.35	0.15			<0.7
Surface hardness (Hv, after 1 day)		56					65	
Radiopacity	+	+	–	+	+			
Adhesive strength (kg/cm^2) enamel dentin	36 38	55 41	23	21	21			

ties of dentin become the index for the physical properties of lining materials, and these properties are especially important in materials used for bases. A wide range of values for compressive strength, a frequently used measure for physical properties, are reported for dentin, i.e., from 2,400 to 3,400 kg/cm^2. The values for glass ionomer cement are closer to that of dentin than are the values for other materials, and some of the glass ionomer products even surpass the compressive strength of dentin. The physical properties of glass ionomer cement can be thought of as special characteristics, and these properties are brought out to their fullest extent when glass ionomer cement is used as a lining material.

Furthermore, it is not enough to measure only the final value of a static strength such as compressive strength to evaluate the physical properties of lining materials; the proportional limit of the process up until the hardened substance breaks and Young's ratio should also be used. In any case, there are reports that glass ionomer cement also has properties closer to dentin than other materials even in these respects.

2. Good handling properties

In general, the easiest way to improve the mechanical properties of the hardened cement is to increase the proportion of powder when the cement is mixed. Therefore, the amount of powder used during mixing for a liner or base is greater than that used for a luting agent, even with glass ionomer cement. For this reason, it has been said that glass ionomer cement is difficult to mix, and that the setting is rapid and the working time short. On the other hand, due to its thick consistency when mixed, little sticks to the spatula, and it is easy to handle within the time allotted for lining procedures.

Furthermore, the amount of liquid used in the products developed as lining materials is increased because a thin layer is desired. Viscosity is low and adhesion to tooth structure is high to make up for sacrifices in the physical properties, and with the use of syringes and applicators, the cement's handling properties can even be said to be good.

3. Little effect on restorative materials

Restorations are placed with a luting agent between them and the lining or base material, and cavity preparations are filled directly on top of the lining or base. The lining and base materials therefore must not have a negative effect on the restorative materials above them. The mechanical properties of the cement are also important when used with metallic restorations which bear a burden of heavy occlusal forces. Lately, however, esthetics have been emphasized even for molars, and the number of cases

Table 3-3. Properties of restorative glass ionomers

	Fuji II	Fuji II-F	HYBond F	Shofu F	Ketac-Fil	Ketac-Silver	Chemfil II	Compos ite MFR	ISO 7489 Type II
Manufacturer	GC	GC	Shofu	Shofu	ESPE	ESPE	DeTrey		
Major usage	Restorative	Restorative	Restorative	Restorative	Restorative	Restorative	Restorative	Restorative	Restorative
Standard powder:liquid ratio	2.7/1.0	1.8/1.0	2.5/1.0	2.5/1.0	Capsule	Capsule	6.8/1.0		
Initial set	4'00"	2'45"	4'00"	4'00"	3'00"	3'00"			~5'00"
Compressive strength (kg/cm^2)	2060	1550	2347	2313	1968	1700		2000	>1275(125MPa)
Diametral tensile strength (kg/cm^2)	90	102	106						
Solubility (1 day, %)	0.07	0.20	0.15	0.15	0.10	0.12			<0.7
Radiopacity	+	-	-	-	+	+	-		
Adhesive strength (kg/cm^2) enamel dentin	47 44				50	50			

restored with resins has increased. Therefore, lining and base materials must not only have adequate physical properties, but must also not interfere with polymerization of resins. Glass ionomer cement is a material which can be used for such purposes without any of the problems listed above.

Furthermore, since resin restorations have some transparency, the color of the cavity floor is reflected to the surface when the thickness of the resin is less than 1 mm, so the color of the lining material can become a problem. However, it is possible to change the color of glass ionomer cement freely, and lining materials the color of dentin have already become commercially available.

4. Additional requirements

The special characteristics of glass ionomer cement also fulfill all of the additional requirements for lining and base materials, as will be explained in detail in later sections. The additional requirements are: no harmful effect on living tissues such as pulp and dentin; stability of the long-term physical and chemical properties of the hardened cement; radiopacity; and adhesion to dentin.

Restorative Glass Ionomers

The properties of representative commercial products in their set and unset states are

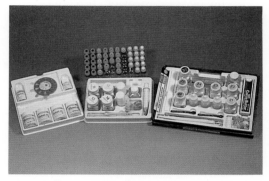

Fig. 3-3. Restorative glass ionomer cement.

shown in Figure 3-3. The following points can be given as requirements for restorative materials (Fig. 3-3).

1. Good physical properties

If a restoration breaks down or deforms, it loses its usefulness as a restoration. Physical strength, however, involves a number of properties, including both compressive and tensile strengths, and when these are examined, the physical properties of glass ionomer cement become evident. In short, this material is strong in compression, but its resistance in tension is low; it is a brittle material.

Glass ionomer cement is therefore best not used on occlusal surfaces or incisal edges where it would be subjected to large mechanical stimuli. Nevertheless, it has been reported in an abrasion experiment (using a toothbrush) that the amount of abrasion caused in this cement was less than that for composite resin.

2. Little dimensional change

Dimensional change occurs primarily at the time of setting, but there are also dimensional changes after that due to moisture or heat. These dimensional changes after setting are related to many clinical problems such as microleakage.

Glass ionomer cement has dimensional changes similar to that of tooth structure. Additionally, it is thought that superior adhesion to tooth structure (such as exhibited by glass ionomer cement) is a factor which decreases dimensional change.

3. Low thermal and electrical conductivity

If a restorative material's conductivity of temperature and electricity is high, the pulp receives needless irritation after restoration of the tooth. Glass ionomer cement is a material with low conductivity.

4. Esthetics

Recently, the esthetic demands on restorative materials have heightened, and the occlusal surface of molars having little to do with outward appearance are even given esthetic considerations.

The color, transparency, and luster of the restorative material must be similar to that of natural enamel, and all of these qualities are found in glass ionomer cement. Depending on how the material is handled, however, problems with esthetics may arise. Good clinical techniques which solve these problems need to be established immediately.

5. Good handling

Ease of handling—from mixing the powder and liquid to placing the cement in the cavity—greatly influences the clinical evaluation of a cement as a restorative material. When glass ionomer cement is mixed for use as a restorative material, it is desirable to use as much powder as possible, because this increases the cement's physical strength. However, since a lesser amount of powder makes the cement easier to use, we have a trade-off situation. Still, we can get the "best of both worlds" by using mechanical mixing and then a syringe to make the filling procedure easier. If we utilize these techniques, glass ionomer cement has great potential as a restorative material.

6. Additional requirements

Other requirements for restorative materials are: that they cause little harm to vital tissues such as pulp and periodontal tissues; adhesion to tooth structure; and radiopacity. These will be discussed in detail in the following sections.

Section 2: Biocompatibility

Yoshinori Ikeda, Tatsuo Ishikawa
Department of Restorative Dentistry
Tokyo Dental College

Introduction

Since the advent of glass polyalkenoate (glass ionomer) cement, the material has become widely used for both nonmetallic restorations and for luting, due to its esthetics and scientific properties. Many improvements have been made since the material was first developed, so the composition of the products presently on the market differs from that of the early products from the 1970s. Glass ionomer cement can now be put into practical use for a wide range of applications: as a restorative material, as a luting cement, and even as a sealant.

Although composite resins are the tooth-colored restorative material most used today, their use still poses some unsolved problems. The effects of procedures (etching) and materials (bonding agents) used in preparation for bonding have not been completely tested, and at the present level of dentistry, a lining or pulp cap should be placed beneath composite resins if consideration is given to the protection of the pulp.

Glass ionomer cement has received much attention lately because of its direct adhesion to tooth structure, an ideal property for a restorative material. Further, glass ionomer cement has come to be used not only as an esthetic restorative material which adheres to tooth structure, but also as an adhesive lining material and as an adhesive artificial dentin (in the "sandwich technique," Fig. 3-4). This new application for glass ionomer cement—as a dentin substitute—could not have been established if

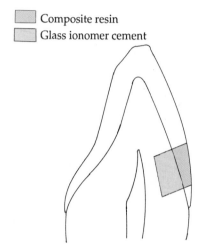

Composite resin
Glass ionomer cement

Fig. 3-4. Sandwich technique.

there were pulpal irritation from the cement itself.

On the whole, the effect of this glass ionomer cement on pulpal tissues is considered to be less than when the cement was first developed, but there has been little systematic research, so we cannot definitely state that the cement is completely safe. In 1983, Tsujimura[F58] studied the effect of glass ionomer cement on pulpal tissue in dog teeth, and Ohashi[F79] then published the results of research studying its effect on human dental pulp in 1986, reaffirming the results of the earlier research indicating that the cement is safe. In this section, I will look mainly at the pathological effects of the cement on dental pulp, and my discussion will be based on the results of the above mentioned research.

What is the Best Tooth-Colored Restorative Material?

It cannot be denied that, at present, composite resins are the tooth-colored restorative material of choice when esthetics must be considered clinically. However, glass ionomer cement has become a frequently used material, specifically being the first choice of many clinicians for restoring cervical abrasion lesions.

A number of different factors can influence the choice between composite resins and glass ionomer cement, but especially with vital teeth, the main factor should be the differences in pulpal irritation (i.e., biocompatibility) between the two materials. About 20 years have passed since composite resins followed acrylic resins into the clinic, and in this period of time many improvements and much research has been done. The biggest improvement was the introduction of etching and the use of bonding agents with the resins. However, when biocompatibility is considered, the problems of etching and bonding have not yet been completely resolved.

Special Characteristics

Adhesion to tooth structure is one of the special characteristics of glass ionomer cement: the cement adheres to both enamel and dentin without even the use of acid etching as is the case with composite resins. This is of great clinical significance because adhesion between the tooth structure and restoration decreases discoloration and microleakage, and reduces the incidence of secondary caries.

Other special characteristics of glass ionomer cement used for restorations, luting, or linings are as follows.

1. Due to very slight differences in the adhesive strengths of glass ionomer cement to enamel and to dentin, a restoration will pull away only slightly from the gingival margin in Class 5 cavities, thus decreasing leakage on the gingival.

2. When a shallow preparation is needed, such as for cavities on the tooth cervix or root surface, the technical problems involved in of layering resin restorative material on the lining material can be eliminated.

3. The adhesive strengths with enamel, dentin and cementum are all relatively stable.

4. Glass ionomers adhere to tooth structure, even without acid etching or other preparatory procedures.

5. Glass ionomer cement exhibits strength close to that of dentin.

Naturally, it is desirable to use glass ionomer cement so as to bring out these advantages in the cases to be treated.

Pulpal Response Toward Glass Ionomer Cement

How Pulpal Responses Were Measured

Pulpal irritation from glass ionomers seems to have decreased since the cement was first marketed. However, as was touched on previously, relatively few studies dealt with pulpal responses early on, and it was not until 1983 that the results of systematic research using dog's dental pulps was reported by Tsujimura. Ohashi, basing his work on Tsujimura's findings, used human dental pulps in his research, and in 1986 reported on the pulpal responses in actual clinical cases.

Tsujimura used various kinds of luting cement, including glass ionomer cement, and experimented on the pulps of dogs, following the ADA tests for dentin and pulps. There are several methods for testing pulpal responses to restorative materials, and both the ADA (American Dental Association), and the FDI (Federation Dentaire International) designate specific experimental methods. For example, observation periods for the ADA are 3 days, 30 days and 60 days, and the experiment is conducted with control groups using materials for which the degree of pulpal response is already known. Zinc oxide eugenol cement is the control causing little pulpal irritation, and silicate cement is the contrasting control causing much irritation.

Table 3-4. Pathologic Responses to Glass Ionomer in the Pulps of Dog Teeth.

Test Groups	Observation Period	Number of Cases	Average Pathologic Points
HG Group	3 days	20	4.4
HY-Bond	30 days	15	4.6
Glass Ionomer	60 days	20	4.7
Zinc Oxide	3 days	20	4.1
Eugenol Cement	30 days	15	4.5
(Neodyne *)	60 days	15	4.5
Silicate Cement	3 days	15	3.9
(MQ Cement)	30 days	15	3.8
	60 days	15	4.5

(Ref.: Tsujimura)

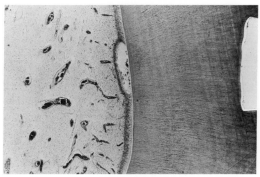

Fig. 3-5. HG Group, short term observation (dog). Region: $\overline{M_1}$. Observation period: 1 day. Pathological state: good. Pathological points: 3. Min. thickness of dentin on cavity floor: 1.4 mm. Suppuration: S-1. Hyperemia S-1, D-2.
(Ref.: Tsujimura)

Tsujimura's research used the same scoring method that this department has used for viewing pathological specimens and evaluating results. Because the various pathological changes appear complex and the extent of the changes vary, a good scoring method must indicate pathological states objectively by assigning point-values to specimens that are otherwise hard to compare. The method here was first used in this department experimentally (1980-1985), and then as a fundamental rule since 1985. Points are given for the extent and degree of both hyperemia and round cell infiltration. That is, definite points are given for the degree of pathological change in the thin layer up until near the enriched-cell region of the pulp, and in the deep layer from deeper regions.

In cases with no pathological pulpal changes recognized at all, or in cases of insignificant injurious pathology of the pulp together with formation of reparative dentin, 5 points are given. In cases of serious pathological pulpal change from which recuperation is not expected, 0 points are given, and conditions between the two are scored in increments of 0.5. When several pathological conditions are seen on the same specimen, the pathological condition with the lowest point score is used.

Dog Pulps

Table 3-4 shows the average scores obtained in the above manner for the glass ionomer luting cement group (*HY-Bond* glass ionomer cement) as well as for the control groups. As seen in this table, the glass ionomer cement had higher scores than the zinc eugenol cement for each observed time period, meaning that the glass ionomer cement produced less pulpal irritation. Figure 3-5 shows the most adversely affected pathological tissue of the HG group. In this pathological specimen, suppuration could be seen near the odontoblast layer, i.e., in the thin layer, and hyperemia could be seen in the relatively deep layer. This was given 3 pathological points. Even in this worst case, then, the extent of the destructive pathological change was small.

These results (from Tsujimura's research) confirmed that glass ionomer cement causes little pulpal irritation in dogs, but this in

Table 3-5. Pathologic responses to glass ionomer cement in the pulps of human teeth.

Experiment Group		Observation Period	Number of Cases	Average Pathologic Points
Indirect Application	Group I	Short	25	4.3
		Long	25	4.5
	Group II	Short	25	4.3
		Long	25	4.5
Pulp exposure		Short	20	1.8

Group I and pulp exposure group : *Fuji Ionomer Type I*
Group II : *Fuji Ionomer Type II*

itself does not necessarily indicate that the material is suitable for humans. Many other aspects are involved in clinical use of the cement, and besides, there is no guarantee that dogs and humans will have the same tissue response.

Human Pulps

Ohashi's research used *Fuji Ionomer*, so a precise comparison to Tsujimura's work cannot be made. Group I used glass ionomer cement for luting and lining, while Group II used restorative glass ionomer cement. In both groups, the cement was placed under the same conditions that would normally occur in the respective clinical application. Also, since restorations are sometimes luted in the clinic without detecting an existing pulp exposure, a group subjected to direct application of the cement onto the dental pulp was also established. This would clarify the pathological changes in the dental pulp and the clinical symptoms from direct contact with the cement.

Table 3-5 shows the pathological changes that resulted. Figure 3-6 is an example of a 5-point score from the short-period for Group I; Figure 3-7 is an example of Group I with a score of 2.5 points, the lowest pathological score in the short-term group, and Figure 3-8 is an example of Group II (long-term group) with the lowest score of 3.5. In the indirect application group, good results—similar to Tsujimura's report—were obtained, but the exposure group in which cement was applied directly had a low score. Figure 3-9 shows pathologic tissue from this exposure group. This group was only observed for a short-term period, but the pathological changes in the specimens make it difficult to contend that there is any tendency for these to heal or recover over the long term.

In his report, Ohashi stated that one cannot contend that glass ionomer cement causes no irritation when applied directly on the pulp, and that there may be almost no repression of the inflammation. It is most accurate to say that direct application of the cement to the pulp may cause some irritation. Still, both Tsujimura's and Ohashi's research support the conclusion that when glass ionomer cement is applied indirectly over the pulp, i.e., with dentin between it and the pulp, there is no tissue irritation whether the material is used as a luting cement, liner or restorative material.

Region: 8
Observation period:
7 days
Clinical state: excellent
Pathological state:
excellent
Pathological points: 3
Min. thickness of dentin
on cavity floor: 2.1 mm
Case of no changes
(Ref. Ohashi)

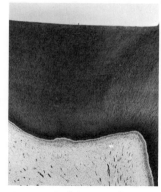

Fig. 3-6. *Fuji Ionomer I* group,
short term observation.

Region: 4
Observation period:
8 days
Clinical state: excellent
Pathological state: good
Pathological points: 2.5
Min. thickness of dentin
on cavity floor:
0.6 mm
Hyperemia:
D-2, round cells
Infiltration: S-1, D-2
(Ref. Ohashi)

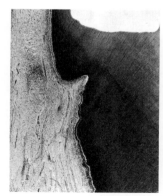

Fig. 3-7. *Fuji Ionomer I* group,
short term observation.

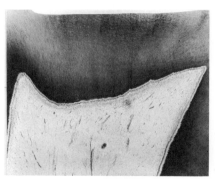

Fig. 3-8. *Fuji Ionomer II* group,
long term observation.
Region: 8
Observation period: 194 days
Clinical state: excellent
Pathological state: excellent
Pathological points: 3.5
Min. thickness of dentin on
cavity floor: 1.8mm
Round cell infiltration: S-1, D-1.
(Ref. Ohashi)

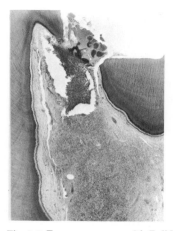

Fig. 3-9. Exposure group with *Fuji Ionomer.*

Region: 5
Observation period: 10 days
Clinical state: excellent
Pathological state: poor
Pathological points: 0
Hyperemia: +++ Round cell infiltration +++
Suppuration: +++
(Ref. Ohashi)

Clinical Symptoms

The task of objectively evaluating clinical symptoms is even more difficult than evaluating pathological specimens. In our department, we have established standards—resembling those used for evaluation of pathological specimens—in an effort to record an individual's perceptions of pain or discomfort. At this point, I would like to examine the clinical results we

obtained for glass ionomer cement using these standards.

In the exposure group from Ohashi's report, 7 out of 50 cases of *Fuji Ionomer Type I*, and 18 out of 20 cases of *Fuji Ionomer Type II* had some symptoms of discomfort. These values are not necessarily all that large, and they may in fact be close to the values for the recent composites that produce relatively little pulpal irritation. However, it cannot be concluded directly from this that glass ionomer cement causes the same degree of clinical discomfort as composite resins.

Ohashi thinks that the cause of the discomfort is not attributable to the glass ionomer cement itself as a cavity lining or restoration, but rather that almost all of the discomfort arises from the irritation caused by the preparation of the cavity. In fact, the discomfort disappeared within 7 days in all but one case; it did not continue for many days. Therefore, it is generally thought that the cement causes no irritation of the dental pulp even clinically. Furthermore, the pathological state of the pulp was good even when symptoms of discomfort did arise, and this discomfort gradually went away.

The above cases were limited to indirect application, but in the pulp exposure group, the condition was somewhat different. In that group, the cement contacted the exposed pulp and mild symptoms of discomfort arose. Some cases showed serious pathological change, so it is necessary to use pulp capping. Glass ionomer cement should not be applied directly when an undetected pulp exposure is suspected: again, in that case it is necessary to use a direct pulp-capping material (Fig. 3-10).

As a Liner or Indirect Pulp Cap

Up to this point, we have dealt mostly with the pathological and the clinical aspects of our topic, but here I would like to examine the possibilities of using glass ionomer cement as a lining material in the sandwich technique.

There are many qualities demanded of a lining material, and the minimal requirement is that it does not irritate the dental pulp. The material should also exhibit a capacity to reverse the damage produced by cavity preparation, and should provide mechanical isolation from external stimuli. Glass ionomer cement satisfies these conditions, as has already been seen. Today there is a glass ionomer cement supplied for use as artificial dentin, but when Ohashi started his research, it was not yet available; there

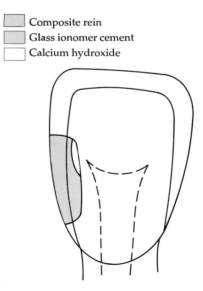

☐ Composite rein
☐ Glass ionomer cement
☐ Calcium hydroxide

Fig. 3-10. Restorative technique for undetected exposure or deep caries.

was only luting and restorative glass ionomer cement. In order to study glass ionomer cement as a lining material, our department conducted research under the same conditions Ohashi used, and then compared the results with research done by Tsunoda[K7] using *Liv Cenera* (a carboxylate cement) and research done by Fujita[K9] using *Palfique Liner* (a lining material with a membrane state).

Other Lining Materials

The research on *Liv Cenera* and *Palfique Liner* was conducted using human dental pulps in a manner similar to Ohashi's. For both lining materials, a composite resin filling was placed over the lining, and the other established conditions were all the same. Both of these materials were developed for use as linings.

The pathological results are as shown in Table 3-6. Figures 3-11 and 3-12 show the differences in pathological changes caused by *Liv Cenera* and *Palfique Liner*, respectively. By comparing cases that were lined with unlined ones, it was found that inflammatory changes were greatly reduced by

Table 3-6. Pathologic states with linings placed.

Experiment Group	Lining Material	Number of Cases	Average Pathologic Points
Durafil	Liv Cenera	31	4.8
	No lining	30	4.4
Palfique	Liner	35	4.7
	No lining	36	4.4

(Ref.: Tsunoda, Fujita) Long period of observation for all.
Note: Pathologic observation based on 5 points for the best state and 0 points for the worst.

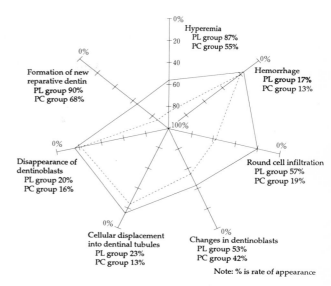

PL group: *Durafil*
PC group: *Liv Cenera + Durafil*
(Ref. Tsunoda)

Fig. 3-11. Observed pathological changes when *Liv Cenera* placed.

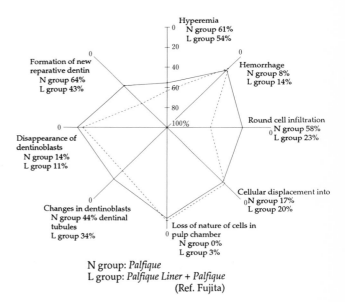

N group: *Palfique*
L group: *Palfique Liner + Palfique*
(Ref. Fujita)

Fig. 3-12. Observed pathological changes when *Palfique Liner* placed.

providing a lining. It can thus be concluded that *Liv Cenera* and *Palfique Liner* are effective liners. However, if these pathological results are compared to those obtained with glass ionomer cement, one finds that glass ionomer cement is less effective than the *Liv Cenera* or *Palfique Liners*, but its effect is somewhat better than the group filled with resin without liners. It can be supposed then that it is possible to isolate stimuli from the composite resin by using glass ionomer cement as a lining. Glass ionomer cement, *Liv Cenera*, and *Palfique Liner* are all either cements or membranes (a slightly different state), and all contain a carboxyl radical in their structure. Also, glass ionomer cement and *Liv Cenera* both include a copolymer of acrylic acid in their composition, and although it may seem plausible to fear stimulation from the low pH of these acids themselves, Wilson[A10] points out that even if the pH is the same, the molecular weight of the organic acids and the inorganic acids are different, so the permeability of the dentin is different. As a result, the pulpal irritation should be small. In any case, tissue irritation by glass ionomer cement has been shown to be slight, and the material meets the requirements of a lining material to a large extent.

Infection

The causes of pulpal irritation are not limited to lining materials, with various factors, as seen in Table 3-7, intertwined in exerting an influence. Among these, the effect of microorganisms within the cavity has received much attention lately as a possible major cause of pulpal irritation. The presence of microorganisms when each of three materials were used is shown in Figure 3-13. As can be seen in the figure, the microorganisms in the group with *Liv Cenera* lining decreased. When the lining was placed with *Liv Cenera*, the rate fell to about half. With *Palfique Liner*, the difference in detection rate was slight, and in the group with the lining, the depth of penetration into the deep layer of dentin on the floor of the cavity became smaller. The detection rate with glass ionomer cement, excluding the pulpal exposure group, was also low. For each material, the incidence of microorganisms was lower when a lining was placed.

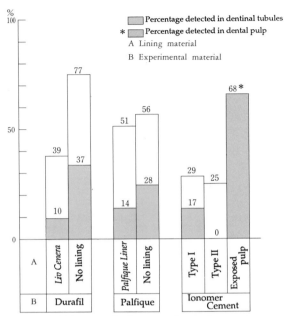

Fig. 3-13. Existence of microorganisms when various lining materials are used (%).

Table 3-7. Causes of pulpal injury from restoring teeth.

Irritation from cavity preparation	Mechanical irritation Thermal irritation Injury to dentinoblast processes Loss of organization in dentinal tubules
Irritation from the restorative material	Penetration of harmful components from the material Adverse effects on dentin by the material Transmission of hot and cold stimulation through the material Transmission of foreign substances through the material
Irritation from microleakage	Penetration of foreign substances Invasion of microorganisms or their toxic products Transmission of hot and cold stimuli
Others	Contamination of cavity walls, remaining pathologic tooth structure, treatment using contaminated materials, accuracy of procedure (techniques of the operator, heat generated), acid treatment, health of the vital tooth (type of tooth, age, extent of disease, whether or not there is pathology)

Fujita has suggested that the reason for this phenomenon when using *Palfique Liner* is that the liner itself has antibacterial properties. *Liv Cenera* or glass ionomer cement may also have antibacterial or bacteriostatic properties, but other explanations—such as the strong acidity of the cement when first applied, or the inadequate space for the development of the bacteria due to the tight contact of the cement to the cavity wall, or some other change in environment affecting the development of the bacteria—are also plausible. The fact that microorganisms are an important factor in pulpal irritation is clear even from Takamori's[K15] report, so the antibacterial or bacteriostatic properties of lining materials is desirable when applying it to the dental pulp. The exact antibacterial and bacteriostatic properties of glass ionomer cement are not entirely clear, but it does seem certain that, when the cement is used, the incidence of microorganisms is low.

Conclusion

As stated above, glass ionomer cement is a restorative material which causes little pathological irritation of the pulp tissues. However, its nonstimulating properties make it suitable only for cases when there is dentin between the cement and the pulp, so if an undetected pulp exposure may occur, glass ionomer cement should not be used. In those cases, a protective material which causes little tissue damage, or a medicament with positive wound healing abilities should be used. It is important to differentiate between cases which need and do not need such protection.

It has been predicted that glass ionomer cement will be used with increasing frequency as both a restorative and lining material. In its present state, the cement can be said to be a useful material for restoring caries.

Section 3: Marginal Seal

Susumu Kawakami, Hirokata Shimokobe
Department of Restorative Dentistry
Hokkaido University Dental School

In recent years, the advent of new bonding techniques has led to a marked improvement in the marginal seal of restorations. However, due to dimensional changes from hot and cold stimulation and from shrinkage at the time of setting, dissolution, and exposure to various harmful factors such as external forces, this marginal seal is difficult to maintain satisfactorily over a long period of time: it eventually deteriorates. This deterioration allows saliva and microorganisms to penetrate into the space between the restorative material or luting agent and the cavity wall, causing hypersensitivity, secondary caries, harmful effects on the pulp, discoloration of the restoration, changes in the color of the dentin, and finally, the loosening or dislodgement of the restoration or prosthesis.

In this section, we will discuss the marginal seal of glass ionomer cement in its various applications as a restorative material, a luting agent, and a sealant. Our discussion is based on research conducted by this department in addition to other references from around the world.

Factors in Marginal Seal

The physical properties which influence the marginal seal obtained by a material include the degree to which it bonds to tooth structure, its shrinkage at the time of setting, water absorption, solubility, and coefficient of thermal expansion. Clinical factors which can lead to the breakdown of the marginal seal include occlusal stresses, abrasion, and thermal stimulation. Furthermore, because cracks and craze lines can appear if the cement is exposed to water or becomes dry when it sets, the prognosis for glass ionomers is also greatly influenced by the application of varnish, the amount of finishing, and the actual techniques used clinically. Each of these factors and how each affects the marginal seal of glass ionomer cement will be discussed in detail in the following passages.

Adhesion

Obviously, the more firmly a restoration adheres to the tooth, the better the marginal seal. To achieve this, the adhesion must withstand various intraoral stresses without breaking down.

Glass ionomers bond chemically to untreated tooth structure, with the bond strength for luting cement to dentin being 12.8-38.0 kgf/cm^2, and the bond strength of restorative glass ionomer to dentin being 28.2-51.0 kgf/cm^2. Similar values can be obtained even for enamel. This bond strength is considerably lower than that obtained between acid-etched enamel and composite resin (150-300 kgf/cm^2), but a stronger bond strength for glass ionomers can be obtained by pretreating the tooth structure with various acids.[D10]

Its chemical bond to tooth structure is extremely advantageous to the marginal seal of glass ionomer cement. However, this bond strength is not high, and it decreases according to the various stresses it receives.

Water Absorption and Solubility

Glass ionomer cement has high water absorption in its initial stage, but once water has been absorbed, the cement becomes stable over a long period. Water absorption during the condensation process, however, decreases the desirable properties of glass ionomer cement and worsens its marginal seal.

The solubility in pure water is 0.1 - 0.3% for restorative glass ionomer and 0.08 - 0.4% for luting cement; this is a considerable improvement over earlier products. However, if the solubility of glass ionomer luting cement is compared to the 0.03% of zinc phosphate cement, it is seen that glass ionomer has a relatively high value. Further improvements in the future, then, are still desirable. The dissolution and erosion of the cement surface of a glass ionomer restoration can even become a factor in the deterioration of its surface characteristics and marginal seal.

Mechanical strength

Glass ionomer cement exhibits more strength from mechanical interlocking forces than from the chemical bond strength itself when resisting occlusal forces. Furthermore, this strength (due to mechanical interlocking forces) is maintained over a long period, and because of this strength, the marginal seal can be preserved. The compressive strength of glass ionomer luting cement is about 1500-2100 kgf/cm[2], a higher value than obtained by zinc phosphate cement.[C46] The strength of restorative glass ionomer, on the other hand, is approximately 1600-2300 kgf/cm[2], considerably lower than the approximately 3150-5000 kgf/cm[2] obtained with amalgam.[C46] Marginal fracture and breakdown of the bond occur when restorative glass ionomer is used in areas with large occlusal forces.

Dimensional Changes

The dimensional changes occurring in dental cement can be divided into three categories: (1) contraction during setting; (2) expansion and contraction due to contact with moisture; and (3) expansion and contraction due to changes in temperature.

These changes in dimension are not much of a problem with luting cement since it is used as a thin film, but for restorative glass ionomer cement, expansion and contraction due to thermal stimulation have a significant effect on the marginal seal. Fortunately, the coefficient of thermal expansion for glass ionomer cement is 13 x 10[-6]/°C, a figure which closely resembles the 11 x 10[-6]/°C of tooth structure, so the expansion and con-

traction probably has little effect as a factor directly causing marginal breakdown.

Other Factors

When moisture contacts glass ionomer cement during setting, the cement's desirable properties decline. In other words, water sensitivity is a problem. Since the setting process is disturbed, the solubility of the margin increases, and this is related to the deterioration of the marginal seal.

Therefore, when using glass ionomer cement, one should take care to minimize contact with moisture. This holds for both luting and restorative glass ionomer cement. An appropriate application of varnish becomes necessary clinically.

Marginal Seal

Marginal Seal in the Literature

In cervical abrasion lesions, Hembree[G4] found that glass ionomer (*ASPA*) restorations had a better marginal seal than composite resins restorations using an enamel bonding system.

Shimokobe et al[G2] prepared Class 5 cavities which extended onto cementum and examined the changes in the gap before and after thermocycling between the restorative material and the cavity wall in vertical sections of cavities filled with either glass ionomer cement (*Fuji Ionomer Type II*) or composite resin using an enamel bonding system. The results showed that whereas the gap at the dentin cavity wall of composite resin enlarged, almost no gap was seen along the entire cavity wall of the glass ionomer cement before or after thermocycling, and there was an extremely favorable marginal seal. Moreover, when a gap was observed, it was not at the junction of the dentin cavity wall and the cement, but in the cement itself—due mostly to breakdown within the cement. Welsh[G11] has similarly reported that glass ionomer cement has a superior marginal seal.

Additionally, Anna[G5] has reported that even after Class 2 cavities in premolars filled

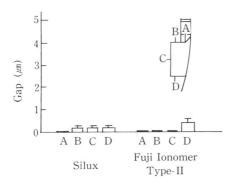

Fig. 3-14. Gap in simple Class 5 restorations for each cavity wall after thermocycling.

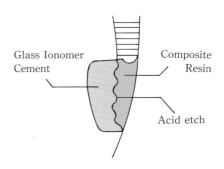

Fig. 3-16. Class 5 restoration using the sandwich technique.

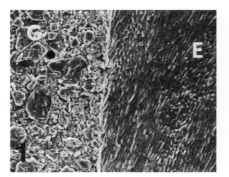

Fig. 3-15. Scanning electron micrographs of Class 5 glass ionomer restoration after thermocycling.

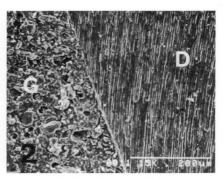

G: Glass ionomer cement
E: Enamel
D: Dentin

with glass ionomer cement (*ASPA, Fuji Ionomer Type II*) were subjected to changes in temperature, only a slight gap occurred at the border of the enamel wall and the cement, or in the cement itself, so the marginal seal obtained by the cement is extremely favorable.

Alperstein[G7] has confirmed that glass ionomer cement in typical Class 5 cavities with walls pretreated with 50% citric acid has only slightly higher microleakage than composite resins using an enamel bonding system or amalgam with cavity varnish. It was deduced that the reason for this leakage was that, compared to cervical abrasion lesions or root surface caries, the shrinkage at setting in typical Class 5 cavities had a greater effect, because the restorative material was surrounded by five walls, and the seal became inferior.

In general, it has been recognized from much research that the marginal seal of glass ionomer cement is favorable when compared to that of composite resins.

Class 5 Cavities

Class 5 cavities were prepared in the buccal surface of extracted human teeth, placing the coronal margin in enamel and the gingival margin in dentin. These preparations were then filled with glass ionomer cement (*Fuji Ionomer Type II*) or light-cured composite resin (*Silux*). Adaptation to the cavity wall was then tested: the changes in the marginal seal before and after thermocycling were examined both by dye penetration and by examining the gap between the cement and the cavity wall in vertical sections.

No gap was found with either the glass ionomer cement or the composite resin before thermocycling, and almost no gap

42

Table 3-8. Degree of dye penetration on the coronal wall in simple Class 5 restorations before and after thermocycling.

Material	Thermal cycling	Number of Specimens	Degree of Dye Penetration			
			0	1	2	3
Silux	before	8	8	0	0	0
	after	11	11	0	0	0
Fuji Ionomer Type II	before	10	10	0	0	0
	after	13	5	7	1	0

Table 3-9. Degree of dye penetration on the gingival wall in simple Class 5 restorations before and after thermocycling.

Material	Thermal cycling	Number of Specimens	Degree of Dye Penetration		
			0	1	2
Silux	before	8	8	0	0
	after	11	7	4	0
Fuji Ionomer Type II	before	10	10	0	0
	after	13	6	7	0

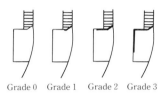

Grade 0 Grade 1 Grade 2 Grade 3

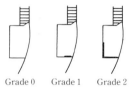

Grade 0 Grade 1 Grade 2

was found even after thermocycling 500 times, so the marginal seal obtained was definitely favorable (Fig. 3-14). Figure 3-14 is a scanning electron micrograph of the coronal and gingival walls of glass ionomer cement after thermocycling. There was no gap between the cement and either the coronal wall or the gingival wall. The cement showed extremely favorable adhesion.

For the composite resin, dye leakage was found only at the gingival cavity wall after thermocycling. For the glass ionomer cement, whereas there was no dye leakage for glass ionomer cement before thermocycling, data (Tables 3-8, 3-9) obtained after thermocycling observed dye penetration along the cavity wall on both the coronal and gingival sides. Nevertheless, the penetration did not advance to the cavity floor.

The reason for dye leakage even when a gap was not observed is as follows. The data obtained in this experiment showed the condition at a single point in time at room temperature. During thermocycling, though the bonding was partially broken down, and with the gap opening and closing with the changes in temperature, the result was that the dye penetrated into the gap.

In any case, about the same marginal seal can be obtained for margins in either enamel

or dentin. This may be because glass ionomer cement bonds effectively to both enamel and dentin.

The Sandwich Technique

For composite resin restorations, a favorable seal cannot be expected when the enamel on the cavity margin is thin or does not exist. For that reason, McLean et al[K4] have recommended the sandwich technique in which the dentin area is restored with glass ionomer cement which bonds to tooth and has little harmful effect on the pulp, and the enamel section is restored in composite resin which is esthetic and has superior abrasion resistance. Using this technique for Class 5 cavities with coronal margins in enamel and gingival margins in root surface, glass ionomer cement was placed within the dentin walls, treated with acid, and composite resin placed following normal techniques, as shown in Figure 3-16.

An experiment on the cement's adaptation to the cavity walls was then conducted. The results after exposure to changes in temperature showed that while no leakage of the dye was found at the coronal margin, a small amount was found between the cement and the resin at the gingival surface, as shown in Table 3-10. Also, a gap was almost never found at either the coronal or gingival surfaces (Fig. 3-17).

The sandwich technique brings out the positive characteristics of glass ionomer cement, and furthermore, the technique can produce an effective marginal seal and be used when the margin of the cavity is in dentin.

Sealants

Resin sealants adhere firmly to tooth structure because of acid etching, and the material is stable with little solubility, so the sealants have the advantage of being maintained over a long period of time. However, increases in the incidence of secondary caries over time have been reported with resin sealants because the resin sometimes fractures and sections are lost. Discoloration and caries underneath the sealant are thought to arise from microleakage.[L14]

The use of glass ionomer cement as a sealant has become increasingly accepted for several reasons: the cement bonds to tooth structure; the acid resistance of the tooth structure can be expected to increase due to absorption of fluoride; and the technique involved is simple. We compared the marginal seal of the glass ionomer sealant recently developed by GC Corp. (*Fuji Ionomer Type III*) to that of commercial resin sealants. When subjected to changes in temperature, no gap was found for the glass ionomer cement despite the fact that a rough surface was exposed. The resin, on the other hand, peeled at the margin, a gap appeared, and the marginal seal deteriorated. It is thought that the glass ionomer's superior performance was due to its bonding molecularly to the enamel, and that compared to the resin, its shrinkage from polymerization condensation and coefficient of thermal expansion are small. It should be added that when we studied the marginal seal in an experiment on toothbrush abrasion, the marginal seal did not deteriorate in either the resin or the glass ionomer cement.

It can therefore be said that when glass ionomer cement is used as a sealant, it is

Table 3-10. Degree of dye penetration on the gingival wall in simple Class 5 restorations using the sandwich technique, before and after thermocycling.

	Thermal cycling	Number of Specimens	Grade of Dye Penetration 0	1	2
Group 1 Silux	before	8	8	0	0
	after	11	7	4	0
Group 2 Lining Cement +Silux	before	10	10	0	0
	after	15	14	1	0
Group 3 Fuji Ionomer Type II F +Silux	before	8	8	0	0
	after	12	12	0	0

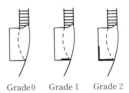

Grade0   Grade 1   Grade 2

superior with respect to marginal seal. However, because sealants are used in the oral cavity on occlusal surfaces which are subject to especially high occlusal forces, it is dangerous to evaluate them solely by their marginal seal. It is necessary to evaluate comprehensively, including long-term clinical observations.

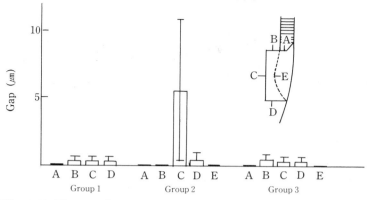

Fig. 3-17. The gap for each cavity wall in Class 5 restorations using the sandwich technique, before and after thermocycling.

Luting Cement

Today, the adaptability of cast items to the cavity preparation has markedly improved because of more accurate casting techniques, but it is still impossible to eliminate the cement line at the margin. For this reason, we still rely on the properties of the cement, the luting agent itself, to maintain the marginal seal. Specifically, the luting agent's strength and solubility are crucial. Glass ionomer cement has superior compressive and tensile strength, and when bonding is added to this, it becomes an extremely effective luting agent. However, as stated before, its solubility is inferior to that of zinc phosphate and carboxylic acid. If the adaptation of the restoration is poor and the cement line large, loss of the restoration may be brought about by water absorption and dissolution.

In an experiment on marginal seal, it was reported that the margin seal obtained with glass ionomer cement was about the same as that of zinc phosphate cement.[G6] However, when varnish was not applied during initial setting, very high leakage and dissolution occurred, and over time, this caused the marginal seal to begin to worsen. Moreover, when the margin is below the gingival border, the application of varnish is not effective, and this causes dissolution by exudate from the periodontal pocket, again leading to the deterioration of the marginal seal.

Marginal Seal in the Clinic

Because glass ionomer cement bonds to dentin, it is very effective in cervical cavities and root surface cavities that have their margins in dentin.

Ziemieckl et al[G16] filled cervical abrasion lesions without retention with composite resin, and when these were observed one year later, a gap was found at the gingival margin in 78% of the cases, and discoloration of the margins was found in 15%. The discoloration of the margins was the result of pigments penetrating between the tooth structure and the resin. Tyas[G14] filled cervical abrasion regions with glass ionomer cement and composite resins, and reported that one year later, discoloration of the margins was seen in the composite resins, but the results with glass ionomer cement were favorable. Even in clinical observations made over four years and six months by Brandau[G8], only 9% of the cases had discolored margins, and no penetration of the discoloration was seen between the cement and the tooth structure.

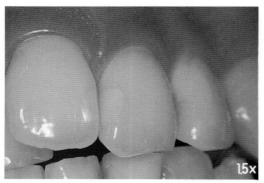

Fig. 3-18. Class 3 glass ionomer restoration in the mesial of the maxillary left central incisor 4 years after placement.

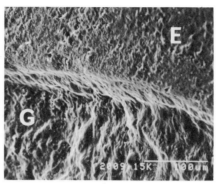

Fig. 3-19. Scanning electron micrograph of the mesial in Fig. 3-18.
    E: enamel
    G: glass ionomer cement

The marginal seal of composite resins deteriorates over time, especially when the margin is in dentin, often causing a gap to appear or the margin to discolor. The marginal seal with glass ionomer cement is superior, and even if dissolution of the margin occurs, discoloration of the margin is seldom seen.

Figure 3-18 shows a glass ionomer restoration done 4 years earlier, and it is passing time favorably without hypersensitivity, margin discoloration, secondary caries, and so on. Figure 3-19 is a scanning electron micrograph of the same case: here, no gap is found between the cement and the enamel, and the marginal seal is good. In spite of the fact that the cement was abraded and a step was formed, there was no discoloration of the marginal region in the oral cavity, and secondary caries were not seen. It is thought that the release of fluoride from the cement participated in the anticariogenic effect.

Conclusion

The maintenance of a marginal seal over a long period of time is extremely important for obtaining a favorable prognosis, avoiding or at least decreasing clinical problems such as the discoloration of margins due to microleakage and secondary caries. Glass ionomer cement causes little pulpal irritation, bonds to tooth structure, and is a superior material with respect to marginal seal. However, as in vitro and in vivo research reports show, it is difficult to say that a perfect marginal seal can be obtained.

Therefore, in order to obtain better marginal seals, it is essential in the clinical use of glass ionomer cement to first understand the properties of the material and learn the correct clinical procedures.

Section 4: Adhesion to Tooth Stucture and Metal

Hirokazu Hashimoto, Yasushi Hibino
Department of Material Science
Meikai University School of Dentistry

Introduction

Zinc phosphate cement, developed by the Rostaining brothers about 100 years ago, has been used as a luting agent for adhering restorations to teeth for a long time. The main component of the powder is zinc oxide, to which 10% oxides (such as magnesium oxide) are added. The powder is then baked and crystalized at 1200°C to 1300°C. The magnesium oxide adjusts the speed of the setting reaction with phosphoric acid, increases the compressive strength of the hardened cement, and helps accelerate crystalization when the powder is manufactured.

The liquid used is an aqueous solution of regular phosphoric acid with aluminum phosphate and zinc phosphate added to adjust the speed of the reaction. The adhesive mechanism of this cement lies not in the adhesiveness of the cement itself, but is due to the mechanical interlocking forces of the cement introduced into the humps and bumps on the interior surface of the prepared cast restoration.

D.C. Smith developed carboxylate cement in 1968, and it is said to adhere to tooth and metal. The powder in this cement is, like that of zinc phosphate cement, zinc oxide, but the liquid is an aqueous solution of polyacrylic acid rather than the aqueous solution of phosphoric acid. It is said that the carboxyl radical ($-COOH^-$) in the polyacrylic acid causes a chelating bond or ionic bond with the calcium ion of the tooth structure, and that there is bonding.

Several years later in 1971, glass ionomer cement was developed by A.D. Wilson and B.E. Kent, and much like carboxylate cement, this cement is also said to have the special property of bonding to tooth structure and metals. The liquid of this cement is the same as carboxylate cement; it is an aqueous solution of a copolymer of acrylic acid and itaconic acid. The powder is the product of melting alumina, silica and calcium fluoride at a high temperature and then grinding it into a powder.

In general, it can be said that the powder is that of silicate cement and that the liquid that of carboxylate acid. This cement therefore has the physical properties and transparency of silicate cement, and moreover, it has the special characteristics of bonding like carboxylate cement, and of not irritating vital pulps. This cement also has the advantage of a coefficient of thermal expansion close to that of tooth structure.

Glass ionomer cement, however, is different from carboxylate cement in that while the chelating bond of the carboxylate cement is the calcium ion of the tooth structure, glass ionomer cement also reacts with the amino acid and the carboxyl radical of the collagen in dentin.

Adhesive resin cement with 4-META monomers added has also been recently developed, and it seems like we have reached an age in which a luting cement can be selected to fit the clinical case. Among all of these cements, glass ionomer produces extremely little irritation of the dental pulp, and similar to carboxylate cement, it bonds chemically to tooth and metal through the mechanism of a setting reaction, as shown in Figure 3-20. Moreover, the cement's physical properties are superior.

Mechanical Strength

Luting cement used for seating crowns, bridges, inlays, and onlays must satisfy the following requirements: a coefficient of thermal expansion appropriate for the tooth or metal (when hot or cold liquids are drunk); the capability of masticating hard and soft foods; the durability to respond to the various conditions present in the oral cavity, which is, for example, moist 24 hours a day; and also, it must be as adhesive, strong, and biologically safe as possible.

A comparison of the physical properties of glass ionomer cement, zinc phosphate cement, and carboxylate cement are shown here. It is clear from the table that the compressive strength of glass ionomer cement is about the same as that of zinc phosphate cement, and its tensile strength is about the same as that of carboxylate cement. Glass ionomer provides the superior properties of both zinc phosphate cement and carboxylate cement, so a cement with considerable bond strength is what one would expect.

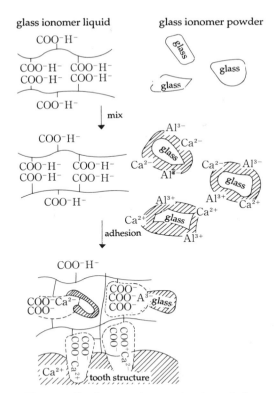

Fig. 3-20. Setting reaction mechanism of glass ionomer cement.

Table 3-11. Physical properties of glass ionomer luting cement.

	glass ionomer A	glass ionomer B	glass ionomer c	zinc phosphate cement	carboxylate cement
powder:liquid ratio	1.8 : 1.g	1.6g : 1.0g	3.4g : 1.0g	1.45g : 0.5mℓ	1.6g : 1.0g
setting time (min)	6.57	6.45	7.27	7.82	7.70
compressive strength (kgf/cm²)	1589	1501	1012	1314	554
tensile strength (kgf/cm²)	63.0	63.0	32.5	37.6	69.1
film thickness (μm)	20.2	19.0	16.8	22.2	20.7
solubility (Wt%)	0.017	0.194	0.073	0.108	0.099

Table 3-12. Changes in compressive strength over time when immersed in water (kgf/cm²).

	Length of immersion (days)					
	1	3	8	15	30	60
glass ionomer cement	1099	1124	1162	1246	1306	1198
zinc phosphate cement	961	1004	1082	1139	1161	1219
carboxylate cement	512	539	546	586	690	633

(Hirano)

Table 3-13. Changes in tensile strength over time when immersed in water (kgf/cm²).

	Length of immersion (days)					
	1	3	8	15	30	60
glass ionomer cement	20.5	20.9	22.3	14.5	11.6	4.1
zinc phosphate cement	1.4	2.8	2.8	4.7	4.7	2.8
carboxylate cement	21.5	21.6	22.4	25.5	22.8	3.3

(Hirano)

Table 3-14. Changes in bond strength over time when immersed in water (kgf/cm²).

	Length of immersion (days)					
	1	3	8	15	30	60
glass ionomer cement	61.5	64.6	70.6	77.4	78.8	75.9
zinc phosphate cement	43.1	45.4	47.4	52.3	56.1	51.4
carboxylate cement	91.3	97.4	107.6	111.4	93.8	92.6

(Hirano)

Table 3-15. Dimensional changes over time when dry or when immersed in water (kgf/cm²).

	Time (days)					
	1	3	8	15	30	60
glass ionomer cement	-5.4 / 0.7	-5.7 / 0.7	-5.9 / 0.7	-6.1 / 0.6	-6.1 / 0.7	-6.3 / 0.7
zinc phosphate cement	-0.9 / -0.1	-1.4 / -0.1	-2.2 / -0.2	-2.5 / -0.2	-2.7 / -0.2	-2.8 / -0.2
carboxylate cement	-5.5 / -0.2	-5.8 / -0.8	-6.4 / -0.8	-6.7 / -0.9	-6.9 / -1.0	-7.2 / -1.1

upper row: dry   lower row: immersed in water   (Hirano)

Tables 3-12 and 3-13 show the changes over time in compressive and tensile strengths of glass ionomer cement immersed in water. Both tables show a tendency for the strength values to increase with time, reaching the highest value at 30 days, then not changing much even after 60 days elapse. These tables only show up to 60 days, but similar results are obtained after 12 more months. Combined with the data from Table 3-11, this information shows that the mechanical strength of glass ionomer cement is superior to that of other cements.

Bonding

As stated previously, bonding by the mechanism shown in Figure 3-21 can also be expected of glass ionomer cement. The hydrogen on the apatite surface of the tooth, hydrogen ions, as well as the metallic ions and organic matter such as the carboxyl radical, the carbonyl radical, amino radical, and imino radical in the collagen form hydrogen bonds to the carboxyl radical in the cement paste, or bonding occurs by the crosslinking reaction of the charged ions, and as a result bond strength increases.

However, when immersed in water, these bonds with tooth structure are easily hydrolyzed by the invasion of water, so the bond strength with tooth structure weakens as time passes. As shown in Table 3-14, glass ionomer cement has a certain degree of bond strength until day 30, but at 60 days, bond strength has weakened to the extent that it is almost nonexistent.

Therefore, observations over a long period of time suggest that one should not expect only chemical bonding, but just like zinc phosphate cement, one should always rely on the interlocking forces exhibited by the superior mechanical strength of the cement itself.

Incidentally, moisture, dimensional change of the cement and humidity in the environment at the time of luting are factors which greatly affect bond strength. Table 3-15 shows dimensional changes in the cement when dry and when in water. Looking at this table, one sees that, at day 1, glass ionomer cement has a change of -5.4% when dry, and +0.7% when wet. After that, there

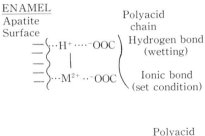

ENAMEL
Apatite
Surface

Polyacid
chain

Hydrogen bond
(wetting)

Ionic bond
(set condition)

Polyacid
chain

Ionic bond

Collagen
backbone

Side-chains

Fig. 3-21. The bonding mechanism of glass ionomer cement. (Phillips: *Skinner's Science of Dental Materials*, 8th ed.)

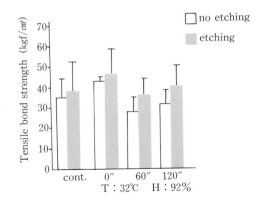

Fig. 3-22. The bond strength of glass ionomer cement to enamel varies with changes in humidity (with reduction). (Higashino)

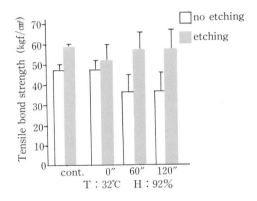

Fig. 3-23. The bond strength of glass ionomer cement to enamel varies with changes in humidity (no reduction). (Higashino)

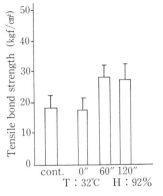

Fig. 3-24. The bond strength of glass ionomer cement to dentin varies with changes in humidity. (Higashino)

are no large changes. One should further note that while carboxylate cement is similar to glass ionomer cement in the dry state, in the wet state, glass ionomer cement expands and carboxylate cement shrinks slightly. Additionally, zinc phosphate cement shows almost no change in either condition.

The dimensional changes of glass ionomer cement can be explained as follows. The cement liquid is made of high molecular substances, and when dry, shrinkage occurs due to the setting, but when wet, expansion from water absorption is even greater than shrinkage from setting. It is thought that this is directly related to bond strength, but because the layer of cement is only a thin film, the effect is extremely small.

An experiment using restorative glass ionomer produced some interesting results, as summarized in Figures 3-22, 3-23, and 3-24. These figures show how the bond strength of the cement with enamel and dentin varied with changes in the moisture in the environment at the time of bonding.

The test subjects listed in Figure 3-22 as "reduction" had 200°m of the surface of the bonding area removed with #600 emery paper, and the "without reduction" in Fig-

50

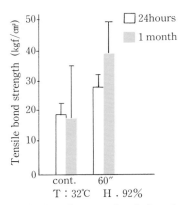

Fig. 3-25. The bond strength of glass ionomer cement to dentin varies with differences in length of preservation. (Higashino)

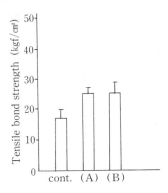

Fig. 3-26. The bond strength of glass ionomer cement to dentin as it varies with smear layer removal. (Higashino)

ure 3-23 was only polished with pumice. Also, a control was bonded at 24°C, with a relative humidity of 50%. According to the results, when there was no etching, those that had set 60 or 120 seconds had a decreased bond strength compared to those which had not set, regardless of whether or not there was reduction. Compared to the control, the bond strength was especially decreased when there was neither reduction nor etching.

In contrast to this, when etching was performed, there was no difference seen in the bond strength either immediately after bonding or when it had set 60 or 120 seconds (Fig. 3-24). The bond strength to dentin immediately after bonding had almost the same value as the control, but those that had set either 60 or 120 seconds showed a slightly higher bond strength.

In addition, Figure 3-25 shows bond strength measured one month after completion of the bonding. The bond strength for that which set 60 seconds was higher than that of the control, even when the stability of bond strength over the long period of one month is considered.

The above results lead one to the following conclusions. High humidity is a factor

decreasing the bond strength of glass ionomer cement, and it is appropriate to regard this as the effect of moisture on the covered surface. However, even if moisture affects the bond strength, lack of both reduction and etching ruin the borders when enamel is the covered surface, and reduction without etching ruins the condensation. The mechanisms of how water affects the bond strength in the above two cases appear to be different. Probably when there is no reduction, the moisture on the surface is bad, and the water adheres locally onto the enamel to be bonded to, thus the bonding of glass ionomer cement to the tooth structure is hindered, and marginal breakdown occurs. But when there is reduction, it is thought that moisture participates in changing the tensile strength of the cement and causing the failure of condensation.

When dentin is the covered surface, the condition of the reduced surface may cause condensation failure, but in contrast to the case of enamel, the strength may increase with moisture. This is because the control group was affected by drying with an air syringe immediately before bonding, and this effect, combined with the porosity of the dentin, caused the cement to become excessively dried. On top of that, when the dentin was bonded to, tensile strength decreased because the cement's moisture was absorbed into the dentin. Bond strength was low, but at both 60 and 120 seconds the excessively dry state disappeared, so it can be supposed that the bond strength in this case is higher than the control's for that reason.

In any case, it is no mistake that the bond strength of glass ionomer cement to dentin increases when under certain environmental temperatures and humidities. This fact should be considered the most significant special characteristic of bonding tooth structure and glass ionomer cement.

Next, the effects of the smear layer, which is produced on the cut surface of the dentin, on the bond strength of glass ionomer cement are shown in Fig. 3-26. That is, the surface of the control to be bonded was exposed with #600 emery paper, and the surface of (A) was treated with a EDTA treatment agent, and the surface of (B) was treated with a polyacrylic acid. The smear layer was removed by using each of the treatments, and as indicated by our results, the bond strength of the glass ionomer cement to dentin became higher.

The bond strength with tooth structure for restorative glass ionomer cement is the same as that for the luting cement, but they are both affected a little by the humidity in the environment at the time of bonding, and by whether or not there is a smear layer. The removal of intervening factors and the removal of humidity elevates bond strength.

Conclusion

Since the development of zinc oxide cement, luting cements have changed to include adhesive carboxylate cement, glass ionomer cement and also resin-type cements which have adhesive monomers. Glass ionomer cement stands out among all of these at the present time because it bonds to tooth structure and metal, and moreover, since it does not irritate living tissues, broad clinical applications can be expected.

As is clear from the discussion above, glass ionomer bonds to tooth structure and metals, but the bond strength decreases over the years in the oral cavity. Consequently, by not depending solely on the adhesive properties of this cement, but by also relying on its the mechanical interlocking forces, glass ionomers can be safely maintained for a long time in the mouth. Because of this, one must always think about possible dislodgement and fear the destruction of the valuable restoration if the cavity or abutment preparations are not made with reasonable retention form. Learning the properties of the cement and dealing with these clinically are important factors in success.

Section 5: Fluoride Release and the Strengthening of Tooth Stucture

Hisanori Komatsu, Hirokata Shimokobe
Department of Restorative Dentistry
University of Hokkaido Dental School

In recent years, glass ionomer cement has been used for various purposes, mostly as a tooth-colored restorative material, but also as a luting agent and a pit and fissure sealant.

Fluoride compounds have been added as flux to the powder of the cement,[B18] and this fluoride is released over time.[F70] The fluoride release causes an elevation in the acid-resistance of the tooth structure,[C6, F41] and fluoride is furthermore thought to produce anticariogenic effects by changing the nature of the plaque surrounding the restoration.[F106] This, along with its bonding to tooth structure and compatibility with dental pulp, have become known as the special characteristics of glass ionomer cement.[F30]

Even if the marginal seal of a glass ionomer restoration breaks down, it can be predicted that the release of fluoride over a long period will suppress secondary caries.[G3,F57,F68] This department continues to conduct basic and clinical research on the movement of fluoride in order to determine how it is released from glass ionomer cement. [F43,90]

In this chapter, we will explain the basics of the anticariogenic properties of fluoride in glass ionomer cement. We will address the action and effects of fluoride, i.e., the release of fluoride from the glass ionomer cement, as well as the acid-resistance properties gained by the enamel.

Fluoride

Caries appear and progress through the interaction of three factors: tooth, bacteria and sugar. Preventive methods include improving eating habits, decreasing cariogenic bacteria, decreasing the number of bacteria adhering to the tooth surface, and increasing the acid-resistance of the tooth.

The following effects of fluoride help prevent caries:[F85]
1. Fluoride decreases the solubility of tooth structure;
2. Fluoride inhibits the growth or metabolism of bacteria;
3. Fluoride changes the adhesive properties of bacteria to tooth.

Basic tooth structure is affected by fluoride. The hydrogen radical of the hydroxyapatite is displaced by fluoride, and fluoroapatite is formed, decreasing solubility toward acid (i.e., elevating acid-resistance). Further, a concentration of fluoride in saliva and plaque, along with fluoride in the pores and minute spaces of the enamel help suppress the dissolution of apatite and promote recalcification.[F87] Fluoride is effective regardless of the age of the patient.[F87]

Studies have also been done on CaF_2, a compound which arises when fluoride, such as NaF, is applied to teeth.[F56,60,61,78] Most of the CaF_2 is washed away by the saliva early on in the oral cavity, but some of this compound remains in the spaces of the tooth structure. This remaining CaF_2 functions as a storehouse, becoming a supply source of fluoride,[F60,61] and it is possible for this CaF_2 to be incorporated into fluoroapatite when phosphate is supplied.[F56] The general perception of CaF_2 has consequently changed lately.

The direct application of fluoride aims to increase fluoride concentration in the enamel, elevate the enamel's acid-resistance, and maintain fluoride concentration above a certain level.[F87] Fluoride rinses and dentrifices containing fluoride are also helpful in maintaining high concentration of fluoride in plaque.

The effectiveness of fluoride is determined by overall caries activity in a given individual, and it is not possible to suppress caries with only fluoride; it is necessary to use other preventive measures jointly to try to decrease the caries activity.[F34]

It has been reported that when plaque is removed from caries on the interproximal surface, the caries are arrested by applying fluoride,[F16] and there are also reports that experimentally, the effect of fluoride is more marked for carious tooth surfaces than for healthy tooth surfaces.[F34] In view of these studies, a method of treating incipient caries using fluoride and not requiring restorations may be on the horizon.

An Anticariogenic Cement

Clinical results show that the incidence of secondary caries in the early silicate cement containing fluoride was low,[F3] and it was also reported that the incidence of interproximal caries of restored teeth was less than when other filling materials were used.[F3] As a result, the effectiveness of the fluoride within the cement was given attention.

The elevation of enamel acid-resistance due to the release of fluoride from the hardened cement has been confirmed through basic research,[F1] and even in artificial caries experiments, suppression of the development of caries has been reported.[F68]

Furthermore, analysis of plaque near the margin of various restorative materials in vivo has suggested that fluoride released in low concentrations from silicate cement had a suppressive action on the metabolism of carbohydrates by bacteria in the plaque.[F7] This result has been confirmed in plaque surrounding restorations over one year after the restorations were placed.

In short, this evidence suggests that secondary caries are repressed by fluoride in cement due to an elevation of the tooth's acid-resistance, and due to the released fluoride changing the nature of the plaque surrounding the restoration. Recently, the promotion of recalcification as an effect of fluoride has been given attention.[F9] When the fluoride is released, it is supplied to the surrounding tooth surface, and caries are repressed.[F77] Then, as the quantity of fluoride released decreases, the elevated acid-resistance of the tooth becomes increasingly important.

Initial Fluoride Release

When the cement is mixed, the surface of the powder is dissolved by the H^+ in the liquid, and the fluoride in the powder is released, along with the positive ions Ca^{2+}, Al^{3+}, Na^+, etc.[F10] During the setting reaction, this fluoride begins to find a place in the matrix, either by itself or as a salt or complex body with positive ions.[F11]

We believe that the fluoride released from the hardened cement is mostly fluoride from the matrix. Initial release is from the fluoride in the surface, and after this, the fluoride from the subsurface of the cement migrates to the surface and is released.[F6, 97] Many points regarding the long-term release of fluoride remain unclear.

Pattern of Fluoride Release

Figure 3-27 shows the changes in amount of fluoride released from hardened cement over time. The concentration of fluoride is measured as the quantity of fluoride released into 10 ml of deionized water from a surface area of 20 mm^2 of test material. This is based on the technique of Ingram,[F5] and it expresses the entire quantity of fluoride, that which reacted with aluminum and also the dissociated fluoride.

The amount of fluoride released is highest for the first 24 hours, beginning with the mixing, and it dramatically decreases over the next 2 or 3 days. Within 1 or 2 weeks, the amount released stabilizes, showing little change, but continues to decrease slowly.

It was confirmed in reports observing fluoride release over one year that the long-term fluoride release of glass ionomer cement resembles that of silicate cement.[F70] It was also concluded from these results that

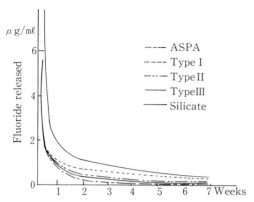

Fig. 3-27. Changes in the amount of fluoride released from hardened cement over time.

Table 3-16. Quantities of fluoride contained in glass ionomer cement powders.

Product	Abbreviation	Manufacturer	quantity of fluoride (%)	powder:liquid ratio (P/L)
Aqua-Cem	Aqua	DE TREY	9.8	7.7
ASPA	ASPA	DE TREY	16.4	1.8
Chem Fil II	Chem	DE TREY	11.3	7.5
Chelon-Fil	Ch-F	ESPE	13.0	3.5
Chelon-Silver	Ch-S	ESPE	6.8	3.8
Ketac-Bond	Ke-B	ESPE	10.2	3.4
Ketac-Cem	Ke-C	ESPE	11.4	3.4
Ketac-Fil	Ke-F	ESPE	14.6	3.0
Fuji Ionomer Type I	Type-I	GC	8.2	1.8
Fuji Ionomer Type II	Type-II	GC	9.9	2.7
Fuji Ionomer Type III	Type-III	GC	11.6	1.2
Ionodent	Iono	Sankin	5.5	5.2
Base Cement	Base	Shofu	9.3	2.6
Glass Ionomer F	GIF	Shofu	9.7	2.6
Hy-Bond Glass Ionomer F	HYF	Shofu	8.5	2.5
HY-Bond Glass Ionomer F	HYC	Shofu	9.6	1.8

the anticariogenic properties of glass ionomer cement were about the same as those of silicate cement.

Differences in Products

The quantity of fluoride contained in the powder of glass ionomer cement is between 5% and 16%, depending on the commercial product (Table 3-16). All glass ionomer products, then, contain a relatively large amount of fluoride, as there is less than 2% fluoride in zinc phosphate cement containing tannin fluoride additive, or in other dental cements. Table 3-16 also shows the powder-to-liquid ratio.

The amount of fluoride released in the first 24 hours after mixing varies greatly between products, but the difference between products becomes small after 4 weeks, so it seems reasonable to assume that there's little difference in the amount of fluoride released over the long term. The bonding state of the fluoride in the powder, however, does differ from product to product.[F41] The powder is made by melting the main components, alumina and silica, with various kinds of flux, and then grinding the result into a powder.[B18] Depending on the melting temperature, some components are only partially melted, and with some, the

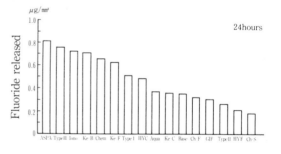

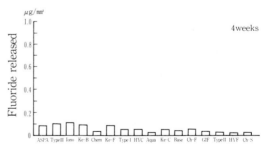

Fig. 3-28. Quantity of fluoride released from glass ionomer cement at 24 hours and 4 weeks.

particles are covered with glass.[F10,88] In *ASPA*, the CaF$_2$ in the powder is covered with glass,[F10] and this may be a key factor in the differences in fluoride release between products.[F41]

The Released Fluoride

The quantity of fluoride released from glass ionomer cement has been discussed above, and the pattern of this release is similar to that of silicate cement. Over the long term, the cement can become a significant source of fluoride. The anticariogenic properties of the fluoride released from glass ionomers can be inferred from studies of silicate cement, as well as from studies of fluoride in general, but the kind of effect fluoride release has on the fluoride in the saliva or plaque has not been studied extensively. Animal experiments have suggested that even a low concentration of 0.38 ppm is effective,[F66] and it is thought that the supply source of fluoride even in glass ionomer cement is significant. Furthermore, when the marginal seal of the restoration starts to break down, the concentration of fluoride is thought to be maintained at a high level due to the limited flow of saliva at the margin.

Fluoride's Strengthening of Tooth Structure

Evaluation of Acid-Resistance

Acid-resistance indicates how much acid the enamel can withstand, and this quantity is clinically related to how easily the caries occur and how quickly they develop. Experimentally, acid-resistance is based on the amount of tooth dissolved when the tooth is immersed in acid for a determined amount of time. Since the amount of dissolution is governed by the type of acid, pH, etc.,[F26] there is no absolute method of evaluation.

When the effects of acid-resistance are studied, acid-resistance is generally expressed as a ratio of the change in the quantity dissolved before (A) and after (B) treatment, to the quantity dissolved before

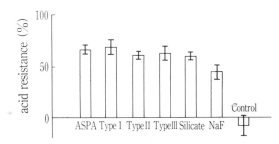

Fig. 3-29. Acid resistance in enamel due to contact with different types of cement or from NaF treatment.

treatment (A-B/A).[F2,29]

Acquiring Acid-Resistance

It is known that when fluoride is contained in a dental material, not only does the acid-resistance of the tooth surface contacting the material increase, but the tooth structure surrounding the material also shows an increase in fluoride due to the fluoride released.[F41] However, because the released fluoride is diluted by saliva in the oral cavity, it is unclear whether acid-resistance can actually be elevated, and if so to what extent. Changes in acid-resistance of the enamel of extracted teeth containing various types of cement is shown in Figure 3-29. Length of contact was one week. The results from a three minute treatment of 2% NaF is shown beside the cement's name. The measurement of the acid-resistance of NaF was conducted 24 hours after application, with the teeth having been stored in water. The acid-resistance test was conducted using an acetic acid buffer solution with a pH of 4 and an immersion time of 20 minutes. The quantity of dissolved Ca was used as an index, and acid-resistance was expressed as the ratio of the change before and after treatment.

The acid-resistance of the enamel increased for all the glass ionomer products, and it was similar to that of silicate cement. Moreover, the glass ionomer cement had values significantly higher than the group treated with 2% NaF.

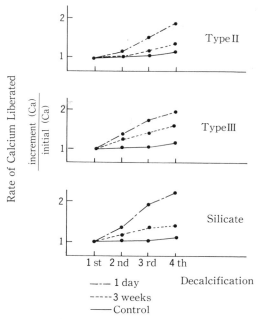

Fig. 3-30. Changes in acid resistance in subsurface enamel for different cements.

Length of Contact

How acid-resistance changes as the length of contact with the cement increases was studied in an experiment on acid-resistance similar to the one discussed above. In the surface layer of enamel, no differences in acid-resistance were found even when the length of contact was changed from 1 day to 1 week or to 3 weeks.[F41] However, when the acid- resistance experiment was conducted after four successive treatments, changes could be found in the acid-resistance of the subsurface enamel. Figure 3-30 shows the changes for each successive decalcification in the experiment, with the amount of dissolved Ca after the first treatment of the cement being equal to 1.

There was not much change in the acid-resistance of surface and subsurface in the control group of untreated cement. When the tooth contacted the cement, the slope of the graph for the first day of contact was more steep than that at 3 weeks, so it is understood that there is a large difference between the surface and the subsurface in how quickly acid-resistance is acquired at this point. At 3 weeks, however, there is a low slope, so the acid-resistance of the subsurface has increased and the strengthening of the tooth has progressed.

Fluoride in the Enamel

The absorption of fluoride from glass ionomer cement (*Fuji Ionomer Type III*) into enamel was studied using extracted teeth.[L28] In order to have a set amount of fluoride in the individual teeth before treatment, the outer surface of the enamel was decalcified with acid and removed, and the surface was polished. Figure 3-31 shows the distribution of fluoride concentration in enamel after one day of contact with the cement. A group treated with 2% NaF for 4 minutes was also studied, and gas chromatography was used to measure the fluoride.[F8] In the group with untreated cement, the fluoride concentration was 300 ppm on the surface, and the concentration in the subsurface was similar. In the group with treated cement, the surface had a high fluoride concentration of 3000 ppm, and the subsurface also had a significant increase in fluoride concentration. Also, the NaF group had a high value in the surface (900 ppm), but the increase of fluoride in the subsurface was hardly noticeable. The enamel contacting the glass ionomer cement already had a significantly higher fluoride concentration at 24 hours than enamel treated with NaF.

Figure 3-32 shows the distribution of the fluoride concentration in enamel according to length of contact with the cement. Here, as contact time with the cement lengthens, fluoride concentration in the enamel increases not only on the surface but also in the subsurface. The amount of fluoride absorbed into the enamel also increases as time passes. In short, glass ionomer cement is capable of supplying fluoride to the enamel it is in contact with, and this process continues over a long period of time. Furthermore, we surmise that the absorbed fluoride is dispersed into the subsurface

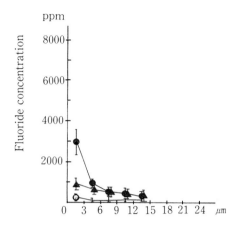

ppm

Depth from enamel surface

Fig. 3-31. Fluoride concentration in the enamel after contact with cement or treatment with NaF before cement treatment (○), after cement treatment (●), after NaF treatment (▲).

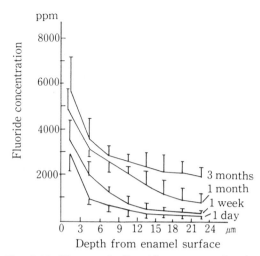

ppm

Depth from enamel surface

Fig. 3-32. Changes in fluoride concentration in enamel according to length of contact with cement.

with the passage of time.

Acid-Resistance

When the fluoride concentration of enamel in contact with glass ionomer cement is studied, both fluoride concentration and the acid-resistance tend to increase. It is generally accepted that the increased acid-resistance is due to the absorption of fluoride, but many points on exactly how this action occurs are still unclear. One plausible explanation is that the decreased solubility is due to the hydroxyapatite shifting to fluoroapatite, a substance which has high acid-resistance.[F87]

Absorption In Vivo

It is known that fluoride which has been absorbed into the enamel from fluoride application flows out of the oral cavity over time.[F60] Therefore, the movement of fluoride taken into enamel from glass ionomer cement was investigated in vivo.[F107] Cement (*Fuji Ionomer Type III*) was placed in contact with the healthy canine or premolar of an adult man for one month, and the fluoride concentration in the enamel was studied

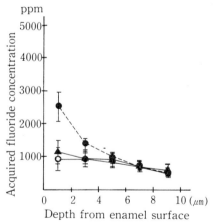

ppm

Depth from enamel surface

Fig. 3-33. Quantity of fluoride taken up from cement. After 1 mo of contact with cement (●), 1 wk after removing cement (▲), and 1 mo after removing cement.

after removal of the cement. Fluoride concentration was measured at one week and one month after the removal of the cement in order to determine the quantity of the outflow of fluoride from the oral cavity. Figure 3-33 shows the results of this study, and indicates the increase in fluoride, i.e., that taken up into the enamel from contact with the cement.

Immediately after removal of the cement, the increased fluoride concentration in the outer surface was 2600 ppm, and fluoride was found to have been absorbed into the subsurface. The fluoride flowed from the glass ionomer cement to the enamel even in the oral cavity, and as the results show, the fluoride concentration in the enamel increased significantly.

An outflow of the absorbed fluoride was found one week later in a portion of the enamel surface. However, since there was almost no change in fluoride concentration one month later, it was determined that there is very little outflow after one week. Moreover, the concentration of fluoride was significantly higher than before application, so it is thought that the effect of fluoride is long term.

This continuing effect of fluoride means increased acid-resistance. Since the fluoride concentration in the enamel increases the longer the cement is in contact with it (Fig. 3-32), it can be predicted that the results of the fluoride absorbed during actual use are greater than the results presented here.

Furthermore, we suggest that the movement of fluoride into fluoroapatite containing CaF_2 is also possible when there is a long length of contact.[F55] In a report about the practical use of glass ionomer as a pit and fissure sealant, it was shown that the anticariogenic effect continued for several years despite a low rate of retention.[L12,13] It is thought that these results show that the strengthening of the tooth by fluoride is valuable even clinically.

Conclusion

The anticariogenic effects of fluoride have been discussed, as have the amount of fluoride contained in glass ionomer cement and the tooth strengthening actions thereby afforded.

It has recently become known that the incidence of secondary caries with this cement is very low clinically,[C53,G8] and that even when the cement is used as a sealant, a high anticariogenic effect can be expected.[L28] The effectiveness of fluoride is largely controlled by the extent of the attack by caries, i.e., the caries activity. From this point on, improved oral hygiene will help to more clearly establish the effectiveness of fluoride in this country. Moreover, when one considers esthetics and the possible necessity of retreatment due to secondary caries, we believe that the use of glass ionomer cement should be actively pursued for its anticariogenic effect.

Section 6: Properties As A Pit And Fissure Sealant

Hirokata Shimokobe
Restorative Dentistry Department
Hokkaido University Dental School

Introduction

Biomaterials have received much attention in recent years, and research continues on them. These materials have been divided into bioactive materials which have positive effects on the living body, and bioinate materials which are stable with respect to the living body and do not have any effect on it.

The author has long held the idea that, especially when it comes to restorative materials, "We should strive for bioactive materials which have positive effects on tooth strengthening and caries prevention, not simply something that fulfills the function of a tooth in the mouth." With this in mind, I have attempted both basic and clinical research on various restorative materials, and here I will take up one of them, glass ionomer cement (in its application as a pit and fissure sealant), and discuss its development.

Motivation for the Development of This Material

Problems with Resin Sealants

Today, resin sealants are used to prevent caries in primary teeth and young permanent teeth, but their success in this application is being reevaluated. Table 3-17 (taken from *Cariology*, by E. Newbrun) shows the requirements for sealants. To what extent do resin sealants really satisfy these demands? It is a fact that resin sealants display several problems, and I would like to point out these problems below.

Figure 3-34 shows a case in which the orifice of the fissure was sealed extremely well in the initial stage, but the enamel walls within the fissure were not sufficiently acid etched, and a small space was left in the fissure because of incomplete adhesion (Fig. 3-35).[L8] Over time in the oral cavity, this kind of condition becomes what is shown as *stage 2* in Figure 3-34. That is, mastication causes marginal breakdown, attrition, and abrasion, and the surface area covering the fissure decreases. As a result, food deposits remain in the broken down area, and the tooth is again threatened by caries. This then becomes what is shown as *stage 3* in the same figure, and as time passes, and oral fluids travel to the deep sections of the fissure, the significance of a sealant ever having been used is lost. Since the solubility of resin is low, and the resin is an extremely stable material in the oral cavity, this condition in *stage 3* continues for a long time, and in the end, the sealant may be destined to fall out.

It has been shown in many clinical records that the incidence of marginal breakdown, dislodgement, and secondary caries, etc., increases with the years.[L11,16,18] Consequently, materials which function only as mechanical seals present problems. Since resin sealants last a long time, periodic examinations are required to determine their prognosis. Resin sealants are therefore extremely effective when the patients remain under the care of a dentist, but for children

Table 3-17. Requirements for Occlusal Sealants (Ernest Newbrun, 1978)

★ Adhesion to enamel for extended periods

★ Simple clinical application

★ Noninjurious to oral tissues

★ Free flowing and capable of entering narrow fissures by capillarity

★ Rapidly polymerized

★ Low solubility in oral fluids

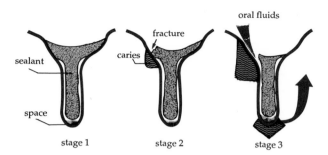

Fig. 3-34. Clinical outcome of resin sealants.

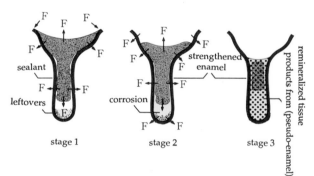

Fig. 3-36. Clinical outcome of sealants based on new concept.

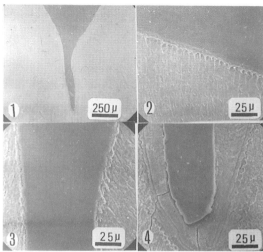

Fig. 3-35. Scanning electron micrograph of a fissure filled with resin sealant *Delton®*.
1. Section of fissure   2. Fissure orifice
3. Central region   4. Floor

Table 3-18. Requirements for pit and fissure sealants. (Shimokobe)

★ Retained in fissure for 1-2 years
★ Simple clinical application
★ Noninjurious to oral tissues
★ Can provide acid resistance (strengthen enamel)
★ Replaced by remineralized tissue

in areas with few dentists, there is room to rethink the matter. When materials are developed, it is always necessary to view their scientific and biological aspects together.

A New Concept for Sealants

The author has drawn up his own blueprints for the ideal sealant, shown in Table 3-18 and Figure 3-36. As shown in Figure 3-36, the condition in this (ideal) initial stage, i.e., *stage 1*, is the same as that for resin sealants, and it would be nice if this condition were maintained for the 1-2 year period of high caries susceptibility following the eruption of the tooth.[L14,15] In this period, an increase in the strength of the tooth is expected because of the fluoride release, and the maturation of the enamel is promoted.[F86]

The process then passes through *stage 2* of the same figure, during which the sealant slowly breaks down and is lost, being replaced by carbonized tissue (pseudoenamel is the proper term). This is *stage 3*. Furthermore, the placement procedure for this material must be simple so that it can be used even in group examinations. Although there are many reports of the elevation of acid-resistance of tooth structure by fluoride[F2,41] and about recalcification, research topics on the formation of pseudoenamel still remain almost untouched. The author views glass ionomer cement as a material with the above possibilities.

J. W. McLean reported trying to use glass ionomer cement as a sealant as early as 1974[L5] and B. Williams et al[L7,12] reported its use in 1976. In both cases, the subsequent

Table 3-19. Composition of test cement.

powder	composition (%) of fluoroalumino silicate glass, average diameter	SiO_2	45
		Al_2O_2	25
		F_2	14
		C_aO, N_aO, P_2O_5	16
	of particles (μm)		1.9
liquid	composition (%) powder: liquid	copolymer of acrylic acid and maleic acid	42
		polycarboxylic acid	11
		H_2O	47
	ratio (g/g)		

Table 3-20. Mechanical properties, test cement.

powder:liquid ratio	1.0
solubility	0.50 (%)
working time	1.0 (min)
setting time	2.5 (min)
compressive strength	1050 ± 60 (24 hrs, kgf/cm²)
tensile strength	3.5×10^4 (24 hrs, kgf/cm²)
adhesive strength (bovine enamel)	33.0 ± 11.4 (kgf/cm²)

Table 3-21. Quantity of fluoride contained in powders of different types of cement (μg/mg).

Cement	Quantity of fluoride	
	Average	Stand. deviation
ASPA®	156	11.2
Type I®	117	7.1
Type II®	113	2.1
Type III®	118	4.6
Silicate	118	6.6
Phosphate	6.5	0.1

*test cement

caries rate was lower than that for resin sealants. However, this research was nothing more than an attempt to substitute restorative cement for resin sealant. Moreover, the glass ionomer cement was divided into soft mix and hard mix, and because of the complicated procedure of first placing the soft mix and then the hard mix, this method is not of much practical use for groups.

In order to develop a glass ionomer cement for sealants which meets the requirements stated above, the author's department began cooperative research with GC Corp. Our initial objectives have not yet been achieved, but a certain amount of success has been obtained with the test *Fuji Ionomer Type III*, and below I would like to introduce the research we have done in this department.[F41,107,L13,20,23,27,28]

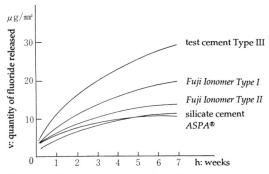

Fig. 3-37. Cumulative quantity of fluoride released from the surface of different types of cement.

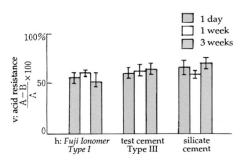

Fig. 3-38. Acid resistance in human enamel after 1 day, 1 week, and 3 weeks covered with different types of cement.

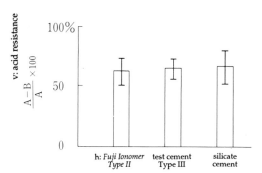

Fig. 3-39. Acid resistance in enamel adjoining different types of cement after 3 weeks.

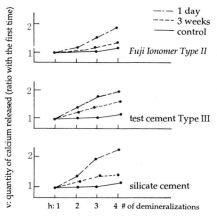

Fig. 3-40. Changes in acid resistance below the surface of human enamel having been covered by different types of cement, after 1 day, 3 weeks.

Properties of *Fuji Ionomer Type III* and Uptake of Released Fluoride

Composition and Properties

Tables 3-19, 3-20, and 3-21 show the composition of the powder and liquid of *Fuji Ionomer Type III*, the properties of the cement, and the amount of fluoride contained in its powder compared to that of other cement.

Amount Released[F41]

Figure 3-37 shows the amount of fluoride released from each type of cement. These values are the result of measuring and

adding the fluoride ion released from a 20 mm^2 surface at each time interval. Even though the amount of fluoride contained in the test *Fuji Ionomer Type III* is not particularly high, the graph shows that the amount of fluoride released is significantly higher than that of other cement.

Acid-Resistance

Figures 3-38 and 3-39 show the acid-resistance of both enamel covered by cement and enamel adjoining cement. The acid-resistance is expressed as the formula $[(A-B)/A] \times 100(\%)$ with the amount of Ca released before cement was applied as A, the amount

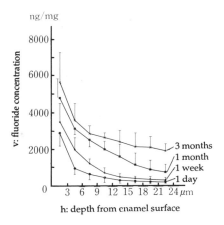

Fig. 3-41. Fluoride concentration in human enamel after 1 day, 1 week, 1 month and 3 months after application of test cement Type III.

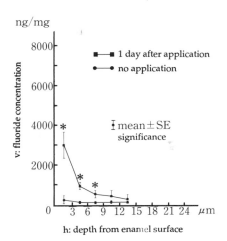

Fig. 3-42. Fluoride concentration in human enamel 1 day after test cement Type III is applied and when it is not applied.

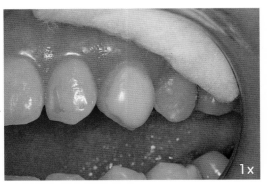

Fig. 3-43. Test cement Type III applied to the labial surface of maxillary right canine.

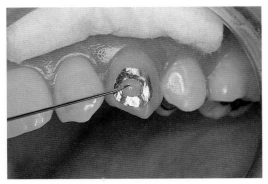

Fig. 3-44. Gathering data from enamel with $HClO_4$ after cement removal.

of Ca after cement was applied as B. It is clear from the same figures that the acid-resistance of the enamel is elevated by applying cement.

Figure 3-40 shows the changes in acid-resistance from the surface of the enamel and into the subsurface. The amount of calcium released during the decalcification treatment with acid was given the value of 1 on the first day after treatment, and the figure shows the rate of change in calcium released during each decalcification treatment from the second time on. The control group did not have cement applied and did not show a large change in the amount of calcium released at each time interval, but in the group which had cement applied, the percentage of released calcium became high-

er each time. When this and the acid-resistance are considered, it supports the theory that acid-resistance was high in the surface of the enamel at the first decalcification treatment. Also, the subsurface showed an acid-resistance close to that of the surface after three weeks.

Uptake of Fluoride into Enamel[L28,F107]

Figure 3-41 shows the amount of fluoride in the enamel after 1 day, 1 week, 1 month, and 3 months following application of the cement in vitro. This is the amount of dissolved fluoride and calcium measured when a set area (2mm²) of enamel surface is affected by 5μL, 1 N, $HClO_4$ continuously for 15 seconds. The figure shows the relationship of the depth from the surface to the concen-

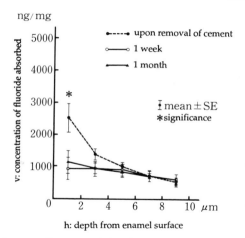

Fig. 3-45. Quantity of absorbed fluoride in the enamel 1 week and 1 month after removal of test cement Type III which had been in place for one month.

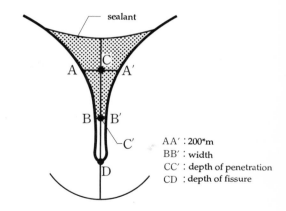

Fig. 3-46. Method of evaluating the penetration of sealant into the fissure.

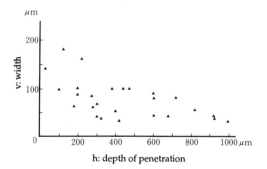

Fig. 3-47. Relationship between depth of penetration and width of the fissure with *Delton®* resin sealant.

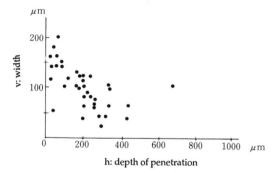

Fig. 3-48. Relationship between depth of penetration and width of the fissure with test cement Type III.

tration of fluoride in enamel. Figure 3-42 shows a comparison with the control (not covered with cement).

The results show that the amount of fluoride in the enamel increased significantly compared to the control group when cement was applied, and that the amount of fluoride also increased significantly by lengthening the period of contact with the cement.

We next investigated the flow of fluoride in the enamel in vivo after cement was removed from the oral cavity of a human (Figs. 3-43, 3-44). The cement was removed 1 month after application, and then the amount of fluoride taken up from the cement was measured immediately after removal,

after one week, and after one month later. These results are shown in Figure 3-45. The amount of fluoride uptake measured immediately after removal was 2,600 ppm in the surface layer, but the amount was decreasing at one week. This means that when the cement is removed, the absorbed fluoride partially dissolves away at first. However, because the values of the graph have subtracted the amount of fluoride contained in the original enamel, it is always about 1000 ppm above that of the control.

The above results suggest that the flow of fluoride when cement is applied is the same whether it is in vivo or in vitro.

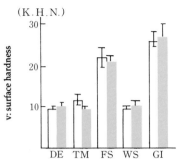

Fig. 3-49. Surface hardness of various sealants.

DE : *Delton®*
TM : *Teethmate S®*
FS : *Fissure Seal®*
WS : *White Sealant®*
GI : test cement Type III
□ : 1 day
▨ : 1 week

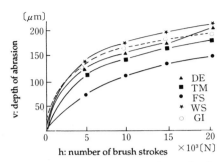

Fig. 3-50. Results of a toothbrush abrasion experiment on various sealants with a load of 200 g.

Penetration and Abrasion Resistance

Penetration into the Fissure[L20]

Standard lines like those in Figure 3-46 were drawn on a sections of extracted human molar which had been sealed with sealants, and the penetration of the sealant was evaluated using the depth of penetration into the fissure and the width of the floor of the fissure. The penetration was divided into a group in which the sealant penetrated only partially down the fissure and a group in which the cement penetrated the full depth of the fissure. If the fissure for the latter group had been deeper, it is possible that the cement may have penetrated further, so the penetration of the former group was compared to the latter. Figures 3-47 and 3-48 show the relationship between the depth of penetration and the width of both the resin sealant and test *Fuji Ionomer Type III* cement. From these graphs it can be seen that the penetration of test *Fuji Ionomer Type III* is inferior to the resin sealants. In order to increase the penetration, it will be necessary to improve the flow and setting time of the cement.

Hardness and Abrasion Resistance

Figure 3-49 shows the hardness of several sealants, and Figure 3-50 shows the results of an abrasion test performed by brushing with a commercial dentifrice and a load of 200g. The hardness of test *Fuji Ionomer Type III* was higher than that of resin sealants, but both showed the same degree of abrasion resistance.

Clinical Results[L13]

Subjects

Children ages five to seven years residing in the jurisdiction of the public health center of a suburb of Sapporo, Japan were chosen as subjects, and the lower first molars of 222 children who were determined to have both right and left healthy teeth were selected. Of these children, 162 had test *Fuji Ionomer Type III* applied to one side while the other side served as a control. The resin sealant *Delton®* was applied to the remaining 60 children. Naturally, consent of the parent was obtained before applying the sealants.

Method of Application

For the test *Fuji Ionomer Type III*, debris was removed from the fissure with an explorer, a prophy brush was used under water irrigation, the tooth was rinsed with water, and dried with air. Following the prescribed procedures, the fissure was filled with cement using a specially manufactured applicator, and varnish was applied. For *Delton®*, the enamel was etched, and the fis-

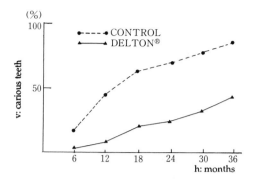

Fig. 3-51. Caries incidence with *Delton®*.

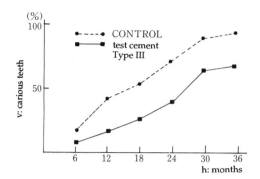

Fig. 3-52. Caries incidence with test cement Type III.

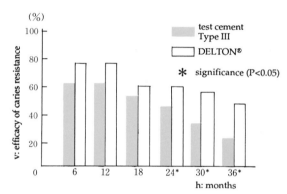

Fig. 3-53. Efficacy of caries resistance with test cement Type III and *Delton®*.

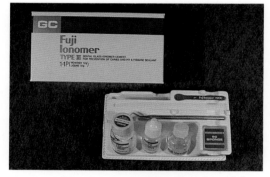

Fig. 3-54. Glass ionomer cement for pit and fissure sealants, *Fuji Ionomer Type III*.

sure was filled following the manufacturer's instructions. Naturally, all procedures were performed under simple isolation.

Method of evaluation

The condition of the teeth was recorded before and after treatment, as well as at each examination, with caries incidence and retention of the sealants evaluated by several examiners. Moreover, photos were taken of the teeth at each examination, and models were made to serve as reference materials for the evaluation.

Clinical Results

Figures 3-51 and 3-52 show the caries incidence over three years for *Delton®* and Fuji cement contrasted with the control. Both materials had decreased caries incidence

compared to the group without any sealants, i.e., the control group, and the Fuji cement had a high value when compared to *Delton®*. Additionally, both groups had a tendency for the caries to increase with the passage of time.

Figure 3-53 shows the effectiveness of the caries resistance as a percentage, according to McCune et al.[14] This is a parameter which expresses the effect of caries resistance, and both materials show effectiveness in caries resistance. The effectiveness of the Fuji cement was inferior to that of the *Delton®*.

As for the retention of the sealants, none of the *Delton®* sealants were lost over the three-year period, but the margins on almost all of the teeth had fractured. On the other hand, almost all of the Fuji cement sealants were lost within six months.

Despite the fact that our test *Fuji Ionomer Type III* was lost in half a year, it showed effective caries resistance. It is thought that this is a very significant effect of the fluoride contained in the cement.

Marketing *Fuji Ionomer Type III*

This material has been developed as a pit and fissure sealant which not only provides a mechanical seal, but also serves as a material with anticariogenic properties, strengthening tooth structure by releasing fluoride. However, the anticariogenic properties of the resin sealants has not yet been reached. To do this, it will be necessary to improve the strength and solubility of the glass ionomer cement material and lengthen its retention period.

In recent years, GC Corp. has marketed *Fuji Ionomer Type III* (Table 3-22, Figure 3-54) with improved properties based on the experimental results above. The authors are conducting clinical experiments with the material,[L23] and a marked increase in its anticariogenic properties and retention rate has been seen in our two-year results. Improvement in the penetration into the fissures has also been achieved.[L27] At present, the authors are hurrying to develop a material which promotes remineralization, and should approach the ideals stated in our opening paragraph.

Conclusion

The development of pit and fissure sealants as bioactive materials was discussed above. It will be necessary from now on to turn our attention to not only this kind of sealant, but also to restorative materials and luting agents which are bioactive, i.e., materials which strengthen teeth and have anticariogenic properties, and also form remineralized tissue between the cavity wall and the restoration. It is necessary to look at today's glass ionomer cement again, and I think that this material should be in active, widespread clinical use today.

Table 3-22. Mechanical properties of *Fuji Ionomer Type III.*

powder:liquid ratio	1.2
solubility	0.15 (%)
working time	1.0 (min)
setting time	2.5 (min)
compressive strength	1600±60 (24hrs, kgf/cm²)
coef. of elasticity	6.0×10^4 (24hrs, kgf/cm²)
adhesive strength (bovine enamel)	45.0±12.0 (kgf/cm²)

CHAPTER IV

HANDLING
GLASS IONOMER
CEMENT

HANDLING GLASS IONOMER CEMENT

Section 1: Theory

Yasuhiko Tsuchitani
Department of Restorative Dentistry
Osaka Dental College

Introduction

The special physical and material properties of glass ionomer cement have been explained in detail in the previous chapters. Generally speaking, glass ionomer cement is a fine powder of aluminosilicate glass containing fluoride and calcium, mixed with a liquid of organic macromolecules. By the attracting charges of the positive ions, Ca^{2+} and Al^{3+}, on the surface of the glass and the negative ions of the liquid, molecules are formed and the cement hardens.

Since this material has a unique system of setting and also an affinity for tooth structure, a broad range of practical applications are possible in the clinic with a little innovation, and the special properties of this cement can then be brought out. Glass ionomer cement was first used as a luting agent, restorative material, and lining cement, and today the cement is also used as a sealant, base, temporary filling, and for buildups.

Guidelines for the effective use of glass ionomer cement to bring out its desirable properties in its various applications will be discussed here.

As a Luting Cement

Glass ionomer cement is used for luting small castings, crowns, and pontics, and this application has even been extended to include orthodontic appliances. This cement has considerable adhesive strength to both untreated dentin and metals, and even when the powder-to-liquid ratio is changed, the cement's properties are not altered much. Nevertheless, it is dangerous to rely exclu-

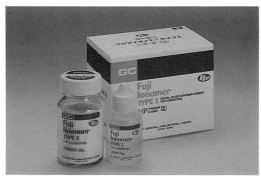

Fig. 4-1. An example of glass ionomer cement, *Fuji Ionomer Type I* (luting, lining).

sively on the cement's adhesive strength for luting, for the material's interlocking forces also play a large role in retaining castings.

The film thickness of glass ionomer cement naturally becomes larger when the powder-to-liquid ratio is large, but when the normal powder-to-liquid ratio is used for luting, film thickness is still smaller than that of zinc phosphate cement. In addition, this cement can be conveniently observed over time (Fig. 4-1) because it is radiopaque.

I would like to enumerate the principles which generally need to be considered when using glass ionomer luting cement.

First, the viscosity of glass ionomer cement is more sensitive to a lowering in the temperature of the mixing pad than is carboxylate cement. It is difficult to change the temperature of mixing paper, and high environmental temperatures are disadvantageous. To increase the cement's interlocking forces, it is advantageous to increase the amount of powder while staying within the

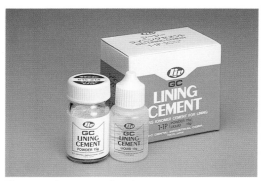

Fig. 4-2. An example of glass ionomer lining cement.

Table 4-1. Tensile strength of glass ionomer cement with 5 commercial resins.

composite resin	ensile strength (kg/cm2)
Silux	42.6 (11.14)
P-30	43.1 (8.25)
Prisma-Fil	42.8 (8.57)
Ful-Fil	49.4 (10.36)
Occlusin	46.3 (8.59)

( ): standard deviation

Average diameter of powder particles was 2.3μm; color was white. It was etched with phosphoric acid 8 minutes after mixing, and bonding agent was applied. (Yoshimura, Junshi: *Jpn J Cons Dent*, Volume 31, no. 4; 1988)

limits of the same viscosity. The cement should be mixed quickly, and moreover thoroughly. Once the mixing has been completed, the cement is immediately applied directly to the surfaces of both the restoration and tooth (cavity preparation), and the restoration is quickly luted in place. If too much time elapses, the film thickness of the cement will suddenly increase.

Cleanliness of the cavity and drying are essential when luting, so contamination with water, saliva, and periodontal fluids should be avoided. Air bubbles are more easily incorporated into this cement than in zinc phosphate, so care must be taken not to do so, and pressure should be applied to the restoration so that it does not float up and become unseated. Furthermore, water absorption increases when the film thickness is large, and this contributes to the breakdown of the cement and the loss of the restoration. There are also reports which say that the bond strength (adhesive strength) of glass ionomer cement decreases some over time, so I would like clinicians to be especially careful when using this cement.

The expressed cement is removed while still soft, and once the cement hardens, varnish is applied to the marginal area and dried lightly with air.

As a Lining

A lining is a thin layer of cement or other material which covers the dentin surface and blocks stimuli from irritating the pulp.

The following are the most demanded qualities of materials used for linings: good handling qualities, little irritation of pulpal tissue, good physical properties even as a thin layer, and good adhesion with the dentin and restorative material. Fortunately, glass ionomer cement is a material which on the whole satisfies these requirements. Moreover, in contrast to zinc oxide cement, it is semitranslucent, so it is good for linings under esthetic restorations, and it is also suitable as a liner under resin restorations as it is able to withstand etching by phosphoric acid.

The working time and initial setting time of this cement used as a lining are shorter than that for other cement, and once the cement is completely mixed, the lining must be placed without hesitation. Care should be taken so that a thick layer is not formed and so that there are not any air bubbles. Once the cement is hard, acid etching can be conducted without any problems.

In the more recently developed lining cement, the pH of the initial set is low (like other glass ionomer cement), but after 24 hours, the pH of some approaches neutrality so the pulpal irritation has also decreased. However, in cases where one section of the cavity is extremely deep or if a pulp exposure is suspected, that section only should be pulp capped (Fig. 4-2).

As a Restorative and Base

A special feature of glass ionomer cement

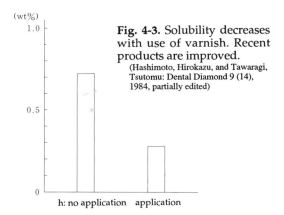

Fig. 4-3. Solubility decreases with use of varnish. Recent products are improved.
(Hashimoto, Hirokazu, and Tawaragi, Tsutomu: Dental Diamond 9 (14), 1984, partially edited)

(wt%)

1.0

0.5

0

h: no application   application

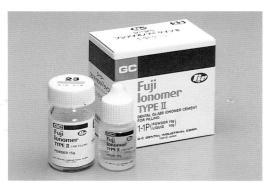

Fig. 4-4. An example of glass ionomer cement *Fuji Ionomer Type II* (restorative, build-ups in vital teeth).

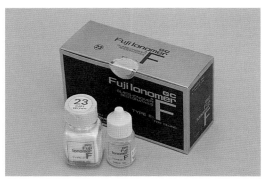

Fig. 4-5. An example of glass ionomer cement *Fuji Ionomer Type II-F* (restorative) fast set.

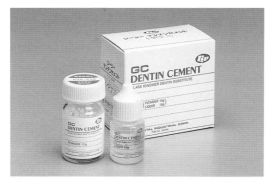

Fig. 4-6. An example of glass ionomer *Dentin Cement* (bases, restorative for primary teeth, restorations in dentin, build-ups of vital teeth).

as a restorative material is that it combines the special properties of liners and of an esthetic restorative materials, so it has a practical application for esthetic restorations in anterior teeth and for restorations in primary teeth. Since glass ionomer cement decreases the occurrence of hypersensitivity and has good marginal seal, it is also often used for the restoration of cervical abrasion lesions and root caries where there are no enamel walls. Recently a new restorative technique called the sandwich technique has been established in which glass ionomer cement is used as a base and composite resin is placed on top. The value of glass ionomer cement in this has been recognized (Table 4-1).

When used as either a restorative or as a base, attention must be paid to the following points: water sensitivity, treatment of the

smear layer, color, placement procedures, contouring anatomy, and finishing.

Glass ionomer cement is particularly sensitive to water during the first 20 minutes after mixing, and if it contacts water, a white spot is formed, causing increased cement solubility and a general worsening of its positive qualities. Therefore, the cavity preparation should be dried, and after placement, varnish should be applied once the initial hardening occurs. Water sensitivity has been greatly diminished in recently improved materials, but it is still not a negligible factor (Fig. 4-3).

When used as a base in the sandwich technique, the cement surface and cavity walls are etched with phosphoric acid once the cement hardens. Bonding agent is then applied, and the resin is placed. The applica-

72

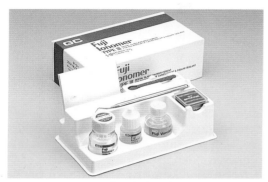

Fig. 4-7. An example of glass ionomer cement *Fuji Ionomer Type III* (pit and fissure sealant).

tion of bonding agent is effective in elevating the adhesiveness of cement and resin. The brightness and opacity generally increase when the cement surface is etched and then rinsed with water, and if the layer of resin in thin, it is possible that the color of the cement will show through too much at the surface. One technique to deal with this is to use resins with rather low transparency (opaque colors).

Incidentally, even though glass ionomer cement is rather opaque when mixed, transparency increases some after placement, and the color also changes. In addition, since the cement paste is viscous, particular attention must be paid so that air bubbles are not trapped in the corners when the restoration is placed. The use of a syringe may be necessary. (See Figures 4-4, 4-5, 4-6.)

If you want to contour the anatomy soon after placement, do it slowly without water, and reapply varnish afterwards. Do only the minimum of contouring necessary on the day of placement. Finishing is done 24 to 48 hours later. At that time, the finishing is done under a stream of water with an ultra-fine diamond point or a white point, and an abrasive strip for interproximal surfaces.

As a Pit and Fissure Sealant

Most pit and fissure sealants are resins, but glass ionomer cement has special features as a sealant that are not found in resins. For example, in contrast to resin, there cannot be a layer of low polymerization due to contact with air on the surface. Also, though there is a tendency for the cement's penetration into the fissure to be somewhat inferior to that of resins, the marginal seal is superior. This seal provides not only a simple physical sealing of the fissure, but also offers effective long term anti-cariogenic properties due to the uptake of fluoride by the enamel. As a result, one of glass ionomer cement's advantages is that even when the sealant is fractured for a short period, the incidence of caries is suppressed.

Points for clinical use will be presented with attention to the special characteristics of this material. First, the tooth is cleansed using a prophy brush under a stream of water, concentrating the polishing on the fissure area. This is necessary to increase adhesive strength between the cement and the tooth. It is not necessary to isolate with a rubber dam, as is the case with resins. Since the working time is short, the mixture is placed quickly after mixing, and only the required amount of the cement paste is taken. There is no need to overfill, and of course acid etching of the tooth is not performed.

There is no formation of a low polymerization layer as in resins, but since water sensitivity becomes a problem, varnish is applied once the cement hardens (Fig. 4-7).

Section 2: Cavity Preparation

Yasuhiko Tsuchitani
Department of Restorative Dentistry
University of Osaka Dental School

Cavity Form

Glass ionomer cement is an esthetic plastic restorative material which has several advantages: it produces little irritation on vital pulps, shows considerable bond strength even with dentin, and increases the acid resistance of the surrounding tooth because of fluoride release from the cement. On the other hand, some problems remain with the cement: water sensitivity is one, and difficulty in adequately resisting occlusal forces is another. It is necessary, therefore, to establish cavity forms which take these advantages and disadvantages into consideration (Fig. 4-8).

Outline Form

Glass ionomer cement provides good marginal seal and secondary caries do not readily occur. Therefore, the outline form of the cavity stops at the extent of the defect or caries, and removal of tooth structure can be kept to a minimum. However, unsupported enamel should not be left in areas subject to external forces. For restoration of cervical abrasion lesions, for which glass ionomer cement is often used, the outline form of the defect is used as the cavity outline form, but sometimes the coronal (enamel) margin is altered (Fig. 4-9).

An area of attention for all cavities with a gingival margin is whether or not the drying of the cavity can be guaranteed. Therefore, if the cavity margin is covered by gingiva or contacts inflamed gingiva, appropriate displacement of the gingiva is suggested (Fig. 4-10). The outline forms for Class 3 and Class 5 cavities for the most part follow the outline forms for composite resin restorations. In any case, it is essential that the outline form be smooth and distinct.

Retention Form

A particular retention form does not need to be consciously provided; in fact, if one is too much of a stickler for the box form, air

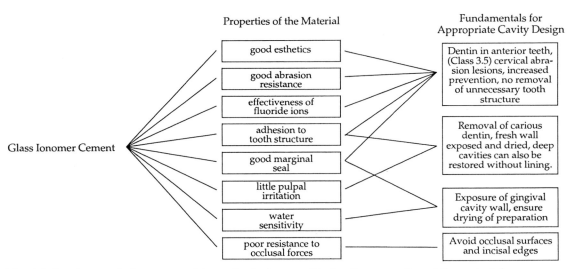

Fig. 4-8. Fundamentals for appropriate cavity design considering the properties of the material.

bubbles will be trapped in the corners. In order to increase adhesiveness with the cement, a fresh dentin surface is exposed as much as possible and any carious dentin is removed. For saucer-shaped cavities, a groove is made in order to help verify the placement, make the placement easier, and prevent fracture of extremely thin margins of cement (Fig. 4-11).

Resistance and Convenience Form

Though glass ionomer cement has great resistance to toothbrush abrasion, it lacks resistance to occlusal forces. Therefore, areas subject to strong occlusal forces should be avoided. Finally, the labial and lingual of Class 3 cavities are sometimes enlarged for convenience when placing the cement.

Type of Margin

It is advantageous to enlarge the surface area to be adhered to, but one must be careful, as margins sometimes fracture when they are extremely thin. Secondary caries in the area of fractured cement does not occur readily. Also, there are not any particular problems with obtuse angles of the same degree as for cavities of composite resins.

Cleansing

The cavity preparation is rinsed with water and dried. Phosphoric acid is not used. Cleansing the cavity with various kinds of organic acids is also being tried at this time. For example, *Dentin Conditioner* (GC Corp.) cleanses the preparation, removes the smear layer, and makes the adhesion of the cement to the dentin surface more reliable. On the other hand, it has also been reported that cleansing with alcohol weakens the adhesion. The exposure of fresh tooth surface and drying are more important than anything else.

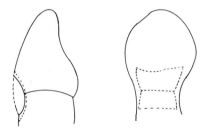

Fig. 4-9. Cervical restoration, considering adhesion and esthetics. (Saito, Sueo: *Dental Outlook*, Vol 54 no. 5, 1979; partially edited).

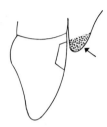

Fig. 4-10. Class 5 cavity restoration and gingivectomy. When the gingival margin is covered with gingiva (healthy or inflamed), and drying the preparation when restoring the tooth is difficult, the gingiva should be displaced (gingivectomy or retraction).

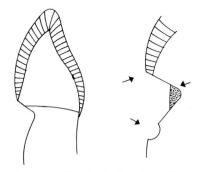

Fig. 4-11. Cervical abrasion. The coronal and gingival cavity walls are modified. Pulp cap only on especially deep lesions. (Katsuyama, Shigeru: *Dental Outlook Clinical Dentistry and Adhesion*, 1983. Fujii, B. et al: *Operative Dentistry Nihon Iji Shimpo*, 1987, partially edited).

Section 3: Measurement and Mixing

Yasuhiko Tsuchitani
University of Osaka Dental School
Department of Restorative Dentistry

Measurement

The properties of glass ionomer cement do not change a great deal even if the powder-to-liquid ratio changes a little. The powder-to-liquid ratio needed to obtain standard viscosity is indicated on the product information sheet, but depending on usage, it may be necessary to alter the powder-to-liquid ratio (Table 4-2).

Essential points for proper measurement are: shaking the bottle of the powder before dispensing the powder, closing the lid immediately after dispensing, not putting the leftover powder back into the jar, and for the liquid, dropping the drops vertically from above the mixing pad (Figs. 4-12, 4-13, 4-14, 4-15).

Table 4-2. Powder-to-liquid ratios and setting times of glass ionomer cement.

		wet mix	standard	dry mix
Fuji Ionomer Type I (luting)	p/l (g/g)	1.4/1.0	1.8/1.0	2.2/1.0
	setting time	7.5	5.5	4.5
Fuji Ionomer Type II (restorative)	p/l (g/g)	2.2/1.0	2.7/1.0	3.2/1.0
	setting time	4.8	4.0	3.0
Fuji Ionomer Type III (sealant)	p/l (g/g)	1.1/1.0	1.2/1.0	1.5/1.0
	setting time	3.3	2.5	2.0
Lining Cement (lining)	p/l (g/g)	1.0/1.0	1.2/1.0	1.5/1.0
	setting time	4.5	4.0	3.5
Dentin Cement (dentin restorative)	p/l (g/g)	1.8/1.0	2.2/1.0	2.6/1.0
	setting time	4.5	3.8	3.0

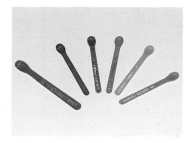

Fig. 4-12. Measuring spoons. The spoon included with the cement is used.

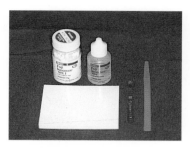

Fig. 4-13. Materials and instruments for measuring and mixing. If one level spoonful of powder to one drop (or 2 drops) of liquid is used, the standard viscosity can be obtained.

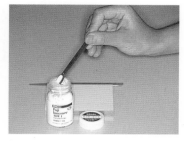

Fig. 4-14. Measuring the cement powder. The bottle is shaken. Powder is scooped with the measuring spoon and leveled off on the lip of the inner lid.

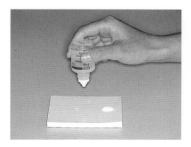

Fig. 4-15. Dispensing the liquid. The bottle is turned upside down, holding it away from the mixing pad, and the drops are released slowly.

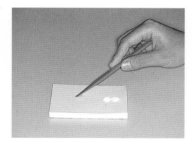

Fig. 4-16. The cement powder is divided into 2 equal parts; the first half of the powder is added to the liquid and mixed until smooth.

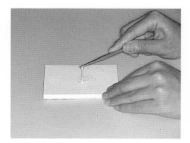

Fig. 4-17. Mixing completed. This is the viscosity for luting inlays. The viscosity is changed depending on the usage.

Mixing

The powder and liquid are placed on the mixing pad and mixed with the plastic spatula provided. The powder is divided into about two parts, with the first portion added to the liquid and mixed uniformly, and then the remaining powder is added and mixed in quickly. The total time to complete mixing about one spoonful of powder is approximately 15 to 20 seconds for sealants and liners, less than 30 seconds for restorative cement, and less than one minute for luting. The cement must be mixed quickly because excess working time is short (especially for the fast-setting types).

Setting time is affected by the temperature of the environment. In recent products, the viscosity of the liquid has been decreased so it is easier to mix, but mixing should not be hurried, as a uniform mixture should be strived for. Restorative cement is mixed as dry as possible (Figs. 4-16, 4-17).

Section 4: Placement and Creating Anatomy

Sueo Saito
Department of Restorative Dentistry
Tokyo Medical and Dental College

Setting Up

Besides choosing the color of the powder and the liquid beforehand, the hand instruments suitable for the type and form of the cavity and its region are set up. In general, the instruments used for placing composite resins are fine (Fig. 4-18), but for cavities in the cervical region, especially saucer-shaped ones, glass ionomer cement placement and carving instruments make the procedure easier. Also, a syringe is always used for shallow, box-form cavities (Figs. 4-20, 4-21).

When the cavity extends into the interproximal, 20 μm metal strips and clips are convenient (Figs. 4-22, 4-23).

Cleansing and Drying

It is fine to cleanse the cavity with the normal method of washing with only water, but *Dentin Conditioner* (GC Corp.), a cavity-cleansing liquid which can cleanse the tooth surface without stimulating the dentinal tubules (Figs. 4-24 through 4-27), is used on painful surfaces, such as those with hyper-

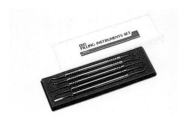

Fig. 4-18. Set of filling instruments for composite resins by GC Corp. This set of 5 instruments can be used for not only large and small cavities and interproximal surfaces, but also for build-ups.

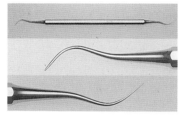

Fig. 4-19. Filling instruments for glass ionomer cement. The tips on both ends are narrow, and thus especially convenient for filling and contouring cervical abrasion lesions.

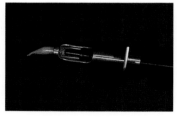

Fig. 4-20. A syringe is always used for box-shaped cavities. Using only hand instruments, air bubbles are trapped, and this may cause loss of the restoration in the future.

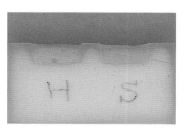

Fig. 4-21. Differences in air bubbles between using hand instruments or syringe for filling. H: hand instruments only. Trapped air bubbles can be seen. S: syringe. Air bubbles do not form easily.

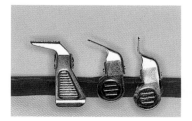

Fig. 4-22. Matrix retainers (clips) A thin tip holds the band better. *Left:* made by Kulzer; *Middle* and *Right:* improved type made by Dentech. There is little pain for the patient if the parts entering into the interproximal are thin, and good retention is achieved with mild pressure from a spring. Also, by rotating the tip around the axis of the tooth, the clip can easily be used in other regions also.

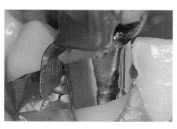

Fig. 4-23. When the restoration is placed using a matrix retainer clip to retain the 20 μm metal matrix, the contact area can be restored without separating the teeth.

sensitivity in the cervical region, or to remove the smear layer of the cavity preparation. Because cavity dryness has a strong effect on adhesion, the preparation is dried carefully, and placement procedures are started while this dry field is maintained. If possible, a syringe with warm air is used for greater effectiveness. Dryers, however, have little air pressure, and are not suitable for drying the tooth surface (Figs. 4-28 through 4-30).

Prompt Placement

Because the bonding mechanism of glass ionomer cement and tooth structure is a chelating bond with the Ca ion of the tooth structure, it is necessary to have the adequately dried tooth structure and the mixed glass ionomer cement contact each other as

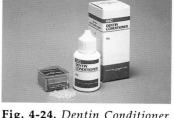

Fig. 4-24. *Dentin Conditioner* (GC Corp.) This liquid for cleansing the tooth has carboxylic acid as its main component and causes little pulpal irritation. It helps with the adhesiveness of the glass ionomer cement.

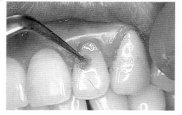

Fig. 4-25. *Dentin Conditioner* is applied for about 10-20 seconds and then rinsed off.

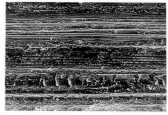

Fig. 4-26. Scanning electron micrograph of the surface of the dentin cavity wall. Smear layer from reducing the tooth covers the dentin (provided by G.C. Research).

Fig. 4-27. Reduced dentin surface after 20 second application of dentin conditioner followed by rinsing. The smear layer has been removed without damaging the tooth fibers.

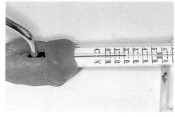

Fig. 4-28. Regular air syringe. Since the temperature does not rise, the tooth can be adequately dried with the air pressure.

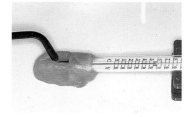

Fig. 4-29. With an air syringe which blows hot air, a temperature of 60°C is reached instantly, so the tooth can be dried well.

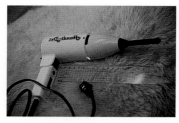

Fig. 4-30. A dryer like this has little air pressure and can not be used satisfactorily for drying moisture, so it is not appropriate for drying the tooth for bonding.

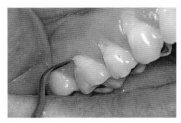

Fig. 4-31. The glass ionomer cement is placed, starting as quickly as possible after mixing.

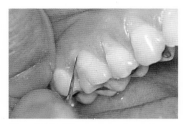

Fig. 4-32. The general contour is completed skillfully while the cement still flows.

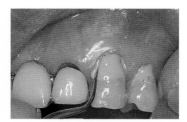

Fig. 4-33. A special instrument for placing glass ionomer cement is useful for shaping the margins.

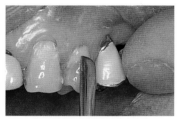

Fig. 4-34. After the fluidity decreases, *Filling Instrument No. 1* (GC Corp.) can be used to easily contour the material.

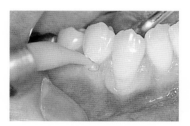

Fig. 4-35. A syringe is used for box-shaped cavities no matter how shallow or small.

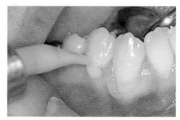

Fig. 4-36. The cavity preparation is filled skillfully, using the syringe so that there are no voids.

soon as possible in order to obtain the best bond. For this reason, both of the above must be done carefully in the initial stages of placement. (Isolation is addressed under a different section.)

The restorative glass ionomer cement is placed in the cavity using a syringe or a special instrument for placing and contouring glass ionomer cement, and the basic anatomy is finished while the cement is still in a fluid state. This is done with the same instrument used for placing and contouring, or with a plastic instrument for composite resins (Figs. 4-31 through 4-34). When a syringe is used, it is pointed into the corners of the cavity and the material is expressed a little at a time, and the cavity floors and cavity walls are filled while withdrawing the syringe from the cavity. The tip of the syringe is used to help seal the perimeter of the cavity, and the cavity is filled so that

there are no voids (Figs. 4-35, 4-36).

All procedures can be performed more quickly and more reliably using a syringe than by placing in increments and contouring, so the use of a syringe is recommended even for saucer-shaped cavities as long as that use is feasible.

Contouring Anatomy

If fluidity disappears while the anatomy is being carved, do not try to create any more anatomy: keep your hands off. Attempts to change the contour after fluidity disappears causes stippling or bumps on the surface. If there is a lack of material, another mix is made quickly and an additional layer added. Extra material should be mixed because addition after the setting has progressed can be a cause of failure and loss due to trapped air bubbles. The following points in particular should be paid attention to.

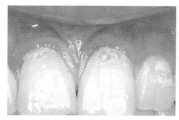

Fig. 4-37. Before restoration. Caries in enamel of the central incisors. The caries will be removed and a saucer-shaped cavity made.

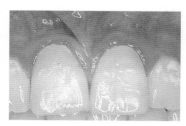

Fig. 4-38. 48 hours after placing glass ionomer cement. There is a slight overfill.

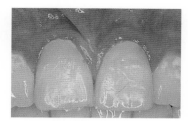

Fig. 4-39. Very little change in contour.

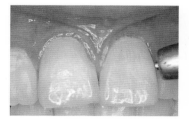

Fig. 4-40. No water sensitivity seen; good prognosis (2 yrs. 8 mos.).

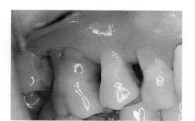

Fig. 4-41. Before restoration. Cervical abrasion lesions in roots of maxillary first molar and first and second premolars. Surface layer will be removed and *Fuji Ionomer Type II* placed in the saucer-shaped cavities.

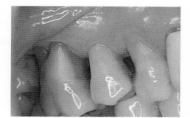

Fig. 4-42. Almost no finishing was done to the maxillary right first molar and first and second premolar after the cement was placed. At 1 yr. 3 mos. the prognosis is good.

1. Cleansing instruments during filling

Glass ionomer cement sticking to the contouring instrument is completely removed each time. When excess cement is stuck on the end of the instrument, it is impossible to take the appropriate amount needed for filling, and the cement also adheres to the surface of the already contoured material or to the cavity margin and it becomes difficult to produce clean anatomy. Furthermore, because of the properties of the cement, water or alcohol must not be applied to the tip of the instrument to prevent the cement paste from sticking to it.

2. "Just filling" is desirable

Anatomy is contoured when it is placed so that the amount to be modified after setting is as small as possible. That is, when the anatomy is completely formed while the material is

fluid, tissue damage from recontouring becomes less, improving overall prognosis (Figs. 4-37 through 4-42).

Contouring of anatomy is completed when there is adequate fluidity because of the reasons given above, and the timing is such that after filling and contouring, one should have to wait only a little bit before the fluidity of the material disappears.

3. Fill one tooth with one mix

There are often many teeth in a row that have cervical abrasion lesions, but you must always fill only one tooth with each mix because, as previously stated, it is essential that the cement contact the tooth at the earliest stage of the setting reaction possible. Also, there is little working time to spare, 2-3 minutes, and the procedure does not take a lot of time even doing one tooth at a time.

Section 5: Isolation

Sueo Saito
Department of Restorative Dentistry
Tokyo Medical and Dental College

Isolation during the placement of glass ionomer cement refers to two separate processes: (1) isolation of the cavity (normal isolation); and (2) isolation of the glass ionomer cement with a covering of varnish (in order to preserve the progression of the chemical reaction of setting).

Number two above is a unique procedure not used for other restorative materials, and since this kind of isolation has a significant effect on the success or failure of the restoration, I would like to refer you to a special section, "Properties of Glass Ionomer Cement You Should Know" (page 96).

Cavity Isolation

Isolation is the same as for other restorative materials, and there are no points which need special mention. It is best, if possible, to use rubber dam isolation. However, when it cannot be used, i.e., when the placement of the rubber dam causes great discomfort for the patient, the clinician should develop another means of adequate isolation. For example, when rubber dam isolation is not suitable for either the tooth or the patient, I have sometimes used two assistants and even two suctions, effectively performing the restorative techniques under conditions drier than with rubber dam isolation. For another example, when restoring the cervical region of mandibular teeth with just one assistant, it is possible to provide adequate isolation until the varnish is applied by retracting the buccal (labial) tissues and continuing suction during placement of the material. Nevertheless, if there is only one technician, the rubber dam will fulfill the function of the other assistant. (In any case, the instruments and materials must be set up properly prior to the procedure.)

This is a very old story, but when glass ionomer cement restorations were in the early stages of development, the following kind of question was received from clinicians, "I properly isolated with a rubber dam and applied varnish, so why did white spots form after the procedure and the phenomenon of water sensitivity occur?" Following the recommended procedures, varnish was not applied after removal of the rubber dam. When the rubber dam was removed from the restorations in the cervical region, the rubber dam scraped off the covering of varnish and when we said that we feared that the protective varnish was peeled off, the clinicians confirmed that that was the case.

To summarize, I think that any method of isolation is fine, as long as good results are obtained. Rubber dam isolation is one such means of obtaining good results.

Finally, some people are concerned about exudate from the cervical region, but in fact, when cervical abrasion lesions are present, most gingival tissues are firm and shallow, and when exudate is measured with an exudate measuring instrument, almost all lesions have a value of 0. Even in the strict sense, if the value is not 0, there will be extremely little exudate, and possibly for that reason, cases showing a lot of water sensitivity are not seen in normal cervical abrasion lesions. Nevertheless, cases showing water sensitivity are seen when there is a lot of exudate and inflammation, so methods of preventing exudate other than just local anesthetic should be considered (Figs. 4-43, 4-44, 4-45). Another technique, similar to that used in placing a filling when there is sudden hemorrhage, is to overfill and then

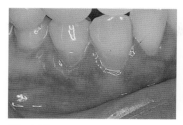

Fig. 4-43

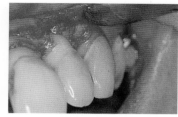

Fig. 4-44

Fig. 4-45

Cases with a lot of exudate in the cervical region, and their prognoses.

Fig. 4-43. Canine and first and second premolars after restoration. With chronic exudative periodontal inflammation with suspected systemic causes, a great deal of exudate may come from the periodontal tissues around the tooth cervix. One thus must pay extra attention to isolation, drying and filling.

Fig. 4-44. After 3 years. No white spots or other signs of water sensitivity seen. Good prognosis.

Fig. 4-45. Restoration of cervical caries on maxillary left lateral incisor, canine, and first premolar before periodontal treatment. Observation about 1 year later when periodontal surgery was performed. A white spot — indicating water sensitivity — can be seen beneath the gingival margin of the canine. With a lot of exudate from the periodontal tissues, not only one must provide adequate drying and proper timing of placement, and should also plan for contouring and finishing the next day. (Essential points are shown in Figs. 4-46 through 4-49.)

Cases in which hemorrhage occurs during filling, and their prognoses.

Fig. 4-46. The filling instrument touched the gingival margin and hemorrhage started. The restoration was placed so as to remove the blood with the restorative material, and varnish was then applied. The patient was sent home like this.

Fig. 4-47. The next day. The area touching the gingival had sensitivity, but it was removed with finishing.

Fig. 4-48. After 1 year, 9 months. This is not a bad result, especially since we thought it would fail.

Fig. 4-49. Results at 7 years, 3 months. There is no particular need to redo the restoration.

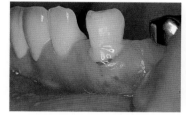

Fig. 4-46

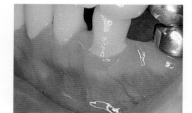

Fig. 4-47

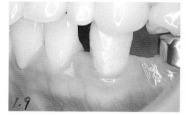

Fig. 4-48

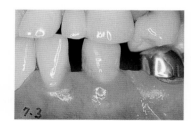

Fig. 4-49

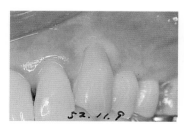

Fig. 4-50. Case finished that had similar hemorrhage.

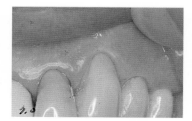

Fig. 4-51. 7 years after restoration.

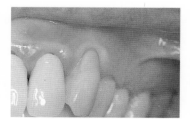

Fig. 4-52. 11 years after restoration. There is some abrasion but no need to redo the restoration.

Note: When there is a lot of exudate or hemorrhage, it is possible to contour and finish the restoration and then send the patient home on the same day if one is using the modern improved glass ionomer cement (*Fuji Ionomer Type II*).

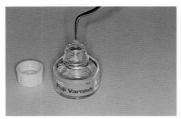

Fig. 4-53. *Fuji Varnish* (GC Corp)

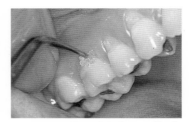

Fig. 4-54. Varnish is applied with a sponge.

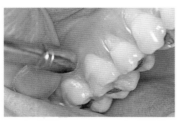

Fig. 4-55. The varnish is dried slowly with light air pressure, but dried adequately so a film is formed.

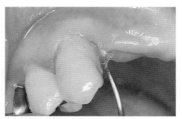

Fig. 4-56. Varnish which has formed a film.

remove the water-sensitive portion after it has set. A good prognosis can be expected using this method (Figs. 4-46 through 4-52).

Varnish Isolation

After the fluidity of the surface of the glass ionomer cement disappears, sufficient varnish is applied to the restoration surface with a soaked sponge, then the surface is dried with air under light pressure, forming a membrane (Figs. 4-53 through 4-56). Varnish is applied as soon as air pressure from the air syringe will not deform the surface, with the earliest possible period being best. The mouth can be rinsed three minutes from the start of mixing, after varnish has been applied. For occlusal surfaces which require adjustment, the adjustment is made after five minutes with light occluding, and varnish is reapplied after adjustment.

These procedures are extremely simple, and while they are not used for other plastic restorative materials, they are extremely important in determining the prognosis of glass ionomer restorations. The importance of isolation by the varnish, its effect, and techniques which enable the clinician to obtain good results even when hemorrhage occurs during the filling procedure will be discussed later.

Many of the fine points of detailed procedures, however, cannot be expressed on paper. Furthermore, even if such procedures were followed step by step, success would not be guaranteed. Instead, if the clinician fully understands the properties of the material she is working with, it will be easy to determine causes and find solutions when problems arise. Then, the fear of poor results should disappear. For these reasons, properties of glass ionomer cement which are closely related to the prognosis are discussed in Section 7 of this chapter, and I would like to refer you to that section here.

Section 6: Contouring Anatomy and Finishing

Sueo Saito
Department of Restorative Dentistry
Tokyo Medical and Dental College

Finishing On or After the Following Day

The final finishing should be done at least one day after the filling procedures so the surface hardness has time to increase. One technique is to contour the basic anatomy using a diamond point (GC) for finishing (Fig. 4-57), and then to finish the surface with *Super Snap*™ disks (Shofu) or some-thing similar. A metal abrasive strip is used for the interproximal surfaces (GC) (Figs. 4-58, 4-59), and the finishing is done so that there are no overhangs (Fig. 4-60). Because the cement is now stable in water, white stone points and silicone points may be used with adequate irrigation. Finishing with polishing pastes, brushes, and rubber cups is avoided because the heat produced may cause craze lines (Figs. 4-61, 4-62).

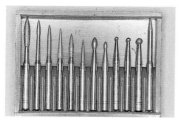

Fig. 4-57. Diamond finishing burs by GC Corp., designed to be used in all areas.

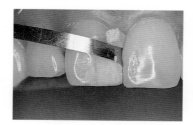

Fig. 4-58. Metal finishing strip slipped between teeth. Improved strips are 30μm thick, so a large space is not needed. A 2μm metal matrix can be used when filling, then finishing strips.

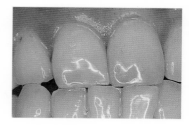

Fig. 4-59. Finishing completed.

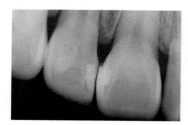

Fig. 4-60. Improved *Fuji Ionomer Type II* shows that there is an overhang on the distal of the central incisor. Correction is possible.

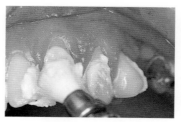

Fig. 4-61. Polishing with paste and a brush is of course avoided during the water-sensitive stage. Polishing after the following day is also avoided.

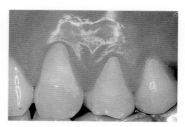

Fig. 4-62. 18 days after restoration. Craze lines from drying appeared more easily here than in other cases, probably from heat during finishing. Next-day finishing must be done under adequate irrigation.

Same-Day Contouring and Finishing

It is possible to do the finishing immediately after filling during the water-sensitive period, i.e., about 15 minutes after the start of the mix. In fact, the anatomy must often be altered in the clinic within 15 minutes even if the final finishing is to be done on a later day. In such a case when the anatomy is adjusted during the water-sensitive period, it is only natural that the procedures are carried out without water irrigation, using instruments that have high cutting ability, such as polishing diamonds. After the occlu-sion is adjusted, varnish is reapplied without rinsing. Even if the restoration is rinsed with water by mistake, there is extremely low water sensitivity with improved *Fuji Ionomer Type II*, so almost no clinical damage occurs (see separate reference). Nevertheless, varnish is applied after finishing. Figure 4-63 shows same-day placement and finishing for a maxillary left canine and first premolar. If the differences in time required are utilized when filling several teeth, contouring anatomy when the restorations are placed can be done relatively easily and efficiently.

Fig. 4-63. Finishing the maxillary left canine and first premolar the same day. As stated in the text, final finishing should be done on or after the following day, but since the water sensitive stage of improved *Fuji Ionomer Type II* is short, it is possible to finish on the same day as filling if there is time available. Especially for several teeth, if the differences in the time of filling are utilized, this can be done with little waiting time.

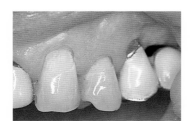

Step 1. Anatomy completed on the canine and first premolar.

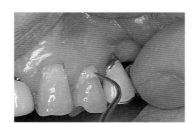

Step 2. Filling the premolar first.

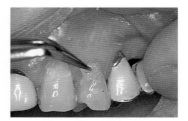

Step 3. Applying varnish.

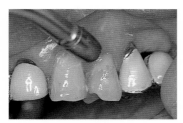

Step 4. Drying, forming a film of varnish.

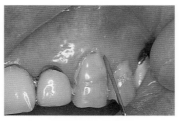

Step 5. Filling the canine.

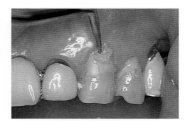

Step 6. Varnish is applied to the canine and dried.

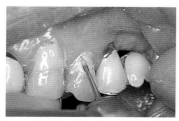

Step 7. 5 minutes after filling the premolar (7 minutes from the start of mixing). Since this is the water sensitive stage, no water is used to create anatomy. A bur that cuts easily is used.

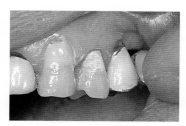

Step 8. Since it is dry, the cut surface is white, but this is not due to water sensitivity.

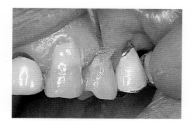

Step 9. Varnish is reapplied.

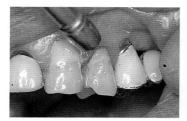

Step 10. A film of varnish is formed again.

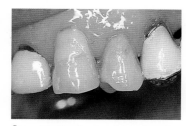

Step 11. 6 minutes has already elapsed since the start of mixing for the canine.

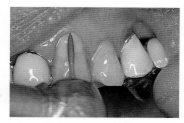

Step 12. Contouring is done as for the premolar.

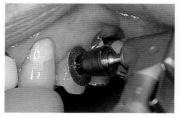

Step 13. After 2-3 minutes, the premolar passes out of the 15-minute water sensitive stage so it can be finished under water.

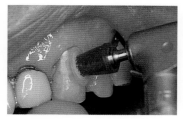

Step 14. After 2-3 minutes, the canine also passes out of the 15 minute water-sensitive stage, so the canine and premolar can be finished together.

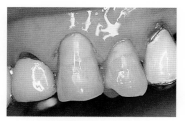

Step 15. Finishing completed. The shade does not match because of drying out from the finishing, but in a few hours they will become the normal shade.

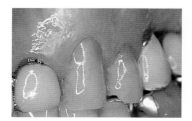

Step 16. Wet appearance 12 months later.

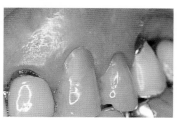

Step 17. White spots from water sensitivity do not appear, even with thorough drying.

Section 7: Properties You Need To Know About Glass Ionomer Cement

Sueo Saito
Department of Restorative Dentistry
Tokyo Medical and Dental College

The Unfortunate Relationship with Water

Whereas composite resin, a tooth-colored restorative material similar to glass ionomer cement, is hydrophobic, glass ionomer cement is a hydrophilic, similar to living things, including teeth. This is a desirable property for restorative dental materials (see separate reference). Furthermore, completely hardened glass ionomer cement can exist in the living body (tooth) and functions as a restoration; it is a hard substance which is extremely stable in liquid and saliva, and the periodontal tissues and tooth have favorable responses to it.

However, when glass ionomer cement is used as a restorative material, it is necessary to "make it set" in the mouth. Though water helps maintain the properties of glass ionomer cement after setting, and is neces-

sary for completing of the setting reaction, it works as an inhibiting factor in the initial stage of the setting reaction. By recognizing this unfortunate relationship between glass ionomer cement and water, it is possible to perform clinical procedures ideally and efficiently and be able to predict the prognosis. Figure 4-64 illustrates the changes in the material's relationship with water, divided into three basic stages of chemical reaction.

Initial Reaction (Water-Sensitive)

At the initial stage of the setting reaction, water interferes in the setting reaction. Although completely set glass ionomer cement is stable in water, our topic here is the period when water from the environment hinders the reaction. That is, water weakens the bonds between molecules, worsening the subsequent properties of the hardened cement, so that when it is dried,

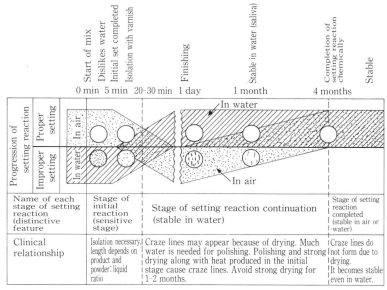

Fig. 4-64. The relationship between water and the setting reaction of glass ionomer cement.

the cement changes to a chalky white state (Figs. 4-65, 4-66). Clinically, this can lead to white spots, wear and tear, craze lines, fractures, discoloration, and staining (Figs. 4-67, 4-68). These may be thought of as symptoms of that problem (Table 4-3).

It is clinically significant that the degree of water sensitivity is greater and extends into deeper areas of the cement earlier in the setting reaction (Fig. 4-69), but decreases as the setting reaction proceeds, and once a certain stage is passed, water sensitivity disappears. The length of the water-sensitive period differs with the product used, the powder-to-liquid ratio, room temperature, and so on.

Reaction Continuation (Stable in Water)

Clinically set glass ionomer cement (i.e., from external appearance) continues to harden in water, and the chemical reaction gradually comes to completion, but the setting reaction continues in water. If the cement is left in the air and dries out before entering the third period (completion of the reaction) craze lines appear because of moisture escape (Fig. 4-70).

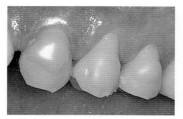

Fig. 4-65. Intraoral water sensitivity experiment (old *Fuji Ionomer*). No isolation was used, and the second premolar was rinsed 5 minutes after mix, the first premolar at 10 minutes, and the canine at 15 minutes. Observed at 24 hours. Even with the same material there are color changes. It is hard to recognize this light water sensitivity.

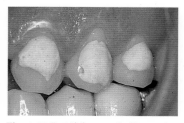

Fig. 4-66. But if the case in Figure 4-65 is dried, white spots are seen. The surface seems to be affected by blowing air.

Table 4-3. Signs of water sensitivity in glass ionomer cement.

- Whiter than normal
- Easily turns chalky white when dried
- Rampant abrasion and attrition
- Craze lines, fractures (Appear especially easily with drying)

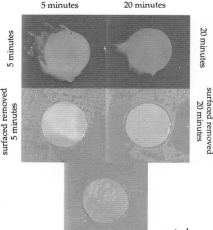

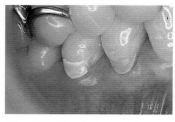

Fig. 4-67. The first premolar was isolated with varnish; no varnish was applied to the second premolar. Observed at 24 hours. The white spot on the second premolar indicates a lot of water sensitivity, but the first premolar shows almost no white spot (no water sensitivity).

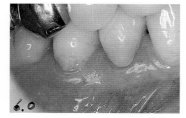

Fig. 4-68. After 6 years. The first premolar had almost no abrasion but the second premolar had a great deal.

Fig. 4-69. Experiment on water sensitivity over time. Removing the surface of the glass ionomer which was water sensitive at 5 minutes still leaves water sensitivity, but at 20 minutes there is much less.

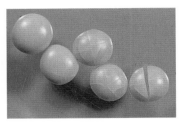

Fig. 4-70. Craze lines appear from drying in the water-stable period. Superficial and fine craze lines also appear (old *Fuji Ionomer Type II*).

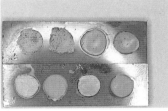
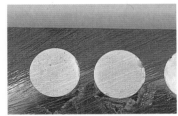

Figs. 4-72, 4-73. Polished and unpolished surfaces of over 100 samples of material preserved in water about 2 years and then left in air for over 3 months. Craze lines are not seen at all. The scratches on the surface are from the polishing instruments.

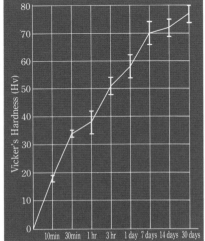

◄ **Fig. 4-71.** Changes in surface hardness over time (old *Fuji Ionomer Type II*).

► **Fig. 4-74.** Changes in compressive strength over time in old *Fuji Ionomer Type II* (GC Research Center).

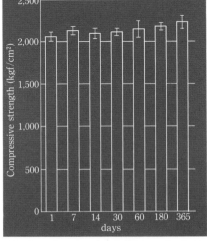

Completion of Chemical Reaction (Stable)

Once the chemical setting reaction has been completed, glass ionomer cement does not readily release moisture, and craze lines caused due to no longer appear (Figs. 4-72, 4-73). That is, glass ionomer cement becomes stable in both air water. The chemical reaction occurs extremely slowly over several months, and the time required for completion is long. This is a property I confirmed with experimental sheets preserved in water for two years and then let dry. Craze lines due to drying do not appear in cases which have set a long time, even in clinical examples.

Relationship With Water in the Clinic

When the above properties are considered clinically, it is clear that attention must be paid to placement, isolation, and application of varnish in order to prevent early-stage water-sensitivity. Furthermore, since finish-ing is done during the water stable period, it is best to avoiding drying when finishing. The setting reaction continues in water (saliva) even after that, and as the values of various properties increase, the cement becomes a stable structure (Fig. 4-74). The completely set cement can then be given a favorable clinical prognosis (separate clinical reference).

Shrinkage

The phenomenon of water-sensitivity is the largest factor negatively affecting the prognosis of glass ionomer cement. Therefore, research on shrinkage during the water-sensitive period is important. Various improvements have been published since about 1983, and the results of studying this water-sensitive period are shown in Figures 4-75 through 4-79.

Figure 4-75 is one part of an experiment which compared the water sensitivity over time of improved and old *Fuji Ionomer Type*

improved *Fuji Ionomer Type II*

old *Fuji Ionomer Type II*

Chelon-Fil

Ketac-Fil

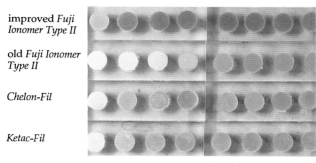

h: time (min)

Fig. 4-75. Changes in water sensitivity over time.

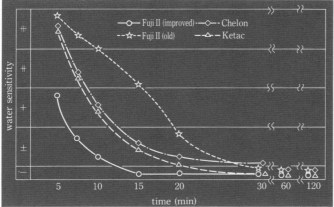

Fig. 4-76. Changes in water sensitivity over time (Saito, Hirota, Akabane).

II, and *Ketac-Fil* and *Chelon-Fil* by ESPE. Each material was put in water 5 to 120 minutes after the start of the mixing, and the degree of water sensitivity was divided into (- to +++) according to the extent of white spots observed on the surface when dried 24 hours later. In this example, the color at 120 minutes showed that the setting reaction had progressed normally, i.e., it could be valued as having had no water sensitivity (-).

The degree of water sensitivity over time can be well understood by comparing these results. For example, the improved *Fuji Ionomer Type II* had about the same color at 10 minutes as it did at 120 minutes, while the old *Fuji Ionomer Type II* was white even at 15 minutes, and finally at 30 minutes the color became the same. In this example, it was concluded that the water-sensitive peri-

od was 10 minutes for the improved type, and 30 minutes for the old type.

ESPE's *Ketac-Fil* and *Chelon-Fil* are said to have a shortened water-sensitive period, but in an experiment in which we (Hirota, Akabane) did a dye penetration test, the penetration for the *Ketac-Fil* product in the capsules was especially large, and it is thought that the water-sensitive period for this product is approximately 20 to 30 minutes.

These results are graphed in Figure 4-76. The old *Fuji Ionomer Type II* had a water-sensitive period of 30 to 60 minutes, with a high degree of water sensitivity during initial setting. Its water sensitivity at 15 minutes was greater than that of *Ketac-Fil* and *Chelon-Fil* at 8 minutes, and the improved *Fuji Ionomer Type II* at 5 minutes. The improved *Fuji*

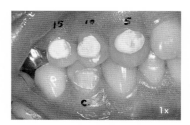

Fig. 4-77. Old *Fuji Ionomer Type II* (GC).

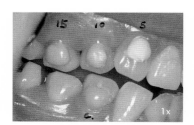

Fig. 4-78. Improved *Fuji Ionomer Type II*.

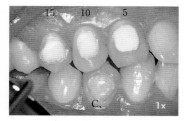

Fig. 4-79. *Chelon-Fil* (ESPE).

Ionomer Type II had a high water sensitivity at 5 minutes but the decrease in water sensitivity was then fast, so at 10 minutes there was water sensitivity, and at 15 minutes, the water-sensitive period was over. The speed of the decrease in water sensitivity in the initial setting period in *Ketac-Fil* and *Chelon-Fil* was fast, but at 15 minutes they remained in the water-sensitive stage, which continues for over 30 minutes.

Figures 4-77, 4-78, and 4-79 show an experiment confirming the water-sensitive times in the oral cavity of old and improved *Fuji Ionomer Type II* and *Chelon-Fil*. From right to left, they were rinsed in water after isolation of 5, 10 and 15 minutes respectively, with controls made by applying varnish to the cement placed on mandibular premolars.

The results were that all of the old *Fuji Ionomer Type II* samples had white spots—water sensitivity. The improved *Fuji Ionomer Type II* had a white spot after 5 minutes, but at 10 minutes almost nothing, and at 15 minutes, showed the same color as the control. *Chelon-Fil* had white spots even at 15 minutes. Also, a white area was seen in the old type at the periphery when the varnish was applied, and a light white spot could be seen also for *Chelon-Fil*, but since almost no white spots could be seen in the improved *Fuji Ionomer Type II*, we submit that this improved type is a superior material, with

the shortest water-sensitive period of all glass ionomer cement tested.

Other Improvements

Improved *Fuji Ionomer Type II* has significantly reduced the problems associated with glass ionomer cement (Table 4-4). Not only was the period of water sensitivity markedly reduced, facilitating same-day contouring and finishing, but the powder particles were made smaller, and the roughness of the surface thereby decreased and other properties improved (Table 4-5). The viscosity of the liquid was also increased, errors in measurement became smaller, and storage qualities improved. In addition, one of the most marked improvements was providing radiopacity, an indispensable feature. Only *Fuji Ionomer* has achieved all of these improvements (see Figs. 4-80 through 4-85, and 4-60).

Efficacy of Varnish

Isolation with varnish is necessary during the water-sensitive stage of glass ionomers. The efficacy of varnish is very striking, as shown in Figures 4-86 through 4-88.

The clinical application of varnish should be early to prevent water sensitivity effects due to the patient's exhalation, but it is better to apply after the cement has set enough so that it is not deformed by pressure of applying the varnish or by the pressure of

Table 4-4. Advantages and problems of glass ionomer cement and the properties of improved glass ionomer cement.

Advantage	Problem	Improved Type(GC Type II, Type I)
Little irritation	Water sensitive	Great improvement
Adhesion to tooth	Shade	Stabilized
Fluoride release	No same-day finishing	Possible (after 15 min.)
Thermal expansion	Powder particle size (largest >30μm)	Finer — (Type II) (largest <30μm)
	Preserves liquid	Great improvement
	Radiolucent	Opacity like enamel
	Viscosity of liquid (1400cP)	Great improvement (600cP)
	Film thickness (25μm)	Great improvement (20μm)—(Type II)

Table 4-5. Comparison of properties.

( ) standard deviation

		Fuji Ionomer Type II (original product)	Fuji Ionomer Type II (improved products)	
powder:liquid ratio (g/g)		2.2/1.0	2.7/1.0	2.2/1.0
setting time (min)		4.5	4.0	4.75
consistency (2.5 kg,mm)		27	29	36
fracture resistance (kgf/cm2)	1 day	1780	2060(120)	1830(80)
	7 days	2040(140)	2130(110)	1940(110)
coef. of elasticity (μ104, kgf/cm2)	1 day	4.84(0.24)	6.64(0.26)	5.79(0.21)
	7 days	5.39(0.26)	7.39(0.49)	6.62(0.30)
adhesive strength (kgf/cm2)	bovine enamel	45(11)	47(8)	45(9)
	bovine dentin	34(8)	44(10)	44(9)
hardness (Hv)	1 day	48	58(3)	49(2)
	7 days	63	70(4)	62(3)
solubility (%)	water	0.40	0.07	0.11
	lactic acid	0.45	0.33	0.36

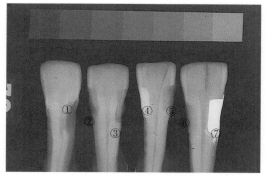

Fig. 4-80. Radiopacity experiment. From *left*: 1. Cavity before filling; 2. Old *Fuji Ionomer Type II*; 3. *HY-Bond Glass Ionomer Cement*; 4. Improved *Fuji Ionomer Type II*; 5. *Ketac-Fil*; 6. *Chelon-Fil*; 7. *Ketac-Silver*.

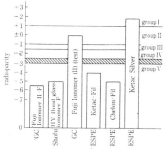

Fig. 4-81. Comparison of radiopacity. Comparison of plugs 2 mm thick. The value of enamel is (-3), and restorations with values less than this may be clinically unclear or misdiagnosed as caries. Except for *Ketac-Silver*, which contains silver, it is clear that the radiolucency of glass ionomer cement is a difficult problem.

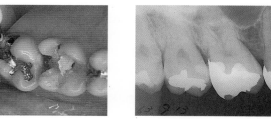

Fig. 4-82.

Fig. 4-83.

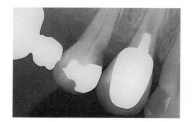

Fig. 4-84.

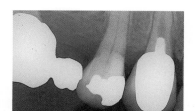

Fig. 4-85.

Fig. 4-82. Deep cavity or mesial surface of the maxillary second molar. Using the cavity of the first molar for access, the second molar was restored with improved *Fuji Ionomer Type II*.

Fig. 4-83. Inlay luted in the maxillary right first molar. Existence of restoration in the mesial of the second molar can be seen clearly.

Fig. 4-84. After cavity preparation for caries on the mesial root surface of the first premolar. (Since the inlay was still good, treatment of only the carious root section was done.)

Fig. 4-85. Restoration with *Fuji Ionomer Type I* (improved). Because it is radiopaque the restored section can easily be observed.

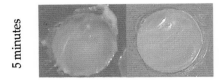

5 minutes

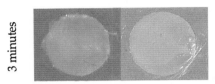

3 minutes

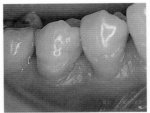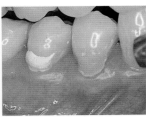

Figs. 4-88, 4-89. Intraoral experiment on the effectiveness of varnish and the differences in the end result. Cervical regions of the right first and second premolars were filled, but only the first premolar had varnish isolation. These are difficult to differentiate by their outward appearance, but when dried, the first premolar, which was covered with varnish, does not change color, while the second premolar becomes a bright white spot. (Refer to Figs. 4-67 and 4-68 for the results of this case.)

Figs. 4-86, 4-87. Experiment on the effectiveness of varnish (old *Fuji Ionomer Type II*). Varnish was applied, and then the samples were immersed in water at 5 minutes (Fig. 4-86) and 3 minutes (Fig. 4-87) after the start of mix. *Left* is the surface as it was and *right* is the surface layer removed. At 5 minutes, water sensitivity was not seen, but at 3 minutes water sensitivity was observed. (Improved *Fuji Ionomer Type II* is not water-sensitive at 3 minutes if varnish is applied.)

air from the syringe. Drying by air is done with low pressure for 10 to 15 seconds, and one should check to make sure that a film has formed completely. For the improved cement, it is even all right to rinse immediately thereafter.

**

Glass ionomer cement must set without being adversely affected by its water sensitivity. Fantastic results can readily be obtained outside the mouth, but sometimes unfavorable symptoms are seen in the clinic. These are usually due to the time limitation of varnish isolation in the oral cavity because the varnish covering peels off due to external forces from the lips and cheeks functioning, and sometimes from food debris.

The shortened water-sensitive period of the improved *Fuji Ionomer Type II* (about 15 minutes) is an extremely significant improvement considering the limited ability of varnish isolation in the oral cavity. Better prognoses with this newly improved product can be expected, along with improved properties, and an expanded range of suitable applications in the general clinic.

Other Factors Worsening Results

Powder-to-liquid ratio, method of measurement, properties, period of water sensitivity, handling, and color

Errors in the powder-to-liquid ratio for cement-type materials affect the properties of the cement, and for glass ionomer cement, this is largely related to the water-sensitive period, significantly affecting overall physical properties and clinical results.

Figure 4-90 shows the changes in water sensitivity in an experiment using the old *Fuji Ionomer Type II*. For example, in a material in which the standard liquid-to-powder ratio is 1:2.2, and the water sensitivity is 30 minutes, if the powder is decreased to 1:1.8, it is still largely water-sensitive 30 minutes after mixing. Also, because the setting time is prolonged (Fig. 4-91), and tear resistance

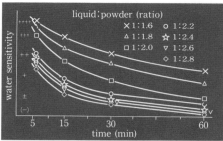

Fig. 4-90. Relationship of powder-to-liquid ratio and water-sensitive period. The more liquid used, the longer the water-sensitive period.

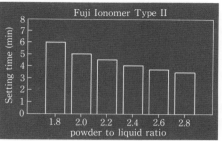

Fig. 4-91. Relationship of powder-to-liquid ratio and setting time. The more liquid used, the longer the setting time.

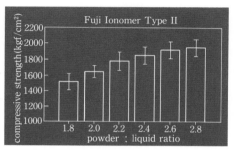

Fig. 4-92. Relationship of powder:liquid ratio and compressive strength. The more liquid used, the lower the compressive strength.

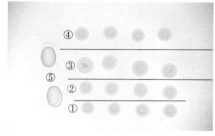

Fig. 4-93. Relationship of the size of the drop of liquid and amount of liquid adhering to the nozzle.
1. New bottle: the first 1-2 drops are small.
2. Nozzle wiped with damped cotton: average size.
3. Liquid adhering to nozzle tip: large. The largest powder: liquid ratio is 1:1.6.
4. Nozzle wiped with dry gauze: smaller than 2, becomes a dry mix.
5. When the amount of powder left in the container decreases, less is measured.

decreases clinically from the standard of approximately 1,750 kgf/cm² to about 1,500 kgf/cm² (Fig. 4-92), the overall properties of become inferior due to the compounded effects of bad conditions. Moreover, since using a lot of liquid improves color and handling in the clinic, this error occurs easily. The tendency to use too much liquid occurs even with the improved *Fuji Ionomer Type II*, though not to the same extent as with other cement. However, since errors in liquid-to-powder ratio are almost always due to errors in measuring the liquid (Figs. 4-93, 4-94), the viscosity of the liquid in improved *Fuji Ionomer Type II* has been lowered.

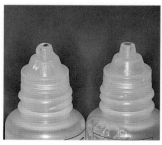

Fig. 4-94. *Right:* liquid adhering to nozzle tip - amount of liquid will increase. *Left:* Wiped with water dampened gauze — appropriate measurement.

SPECIAL NOTE: WHY GLASS IONOMER CEMENT IS POPULAR IN EUROPE AND AMERICA BUT HATED IN JAPAN

When first using glass ionomer cement for restorations, everyone feels that it is a difficult material to work with. This feeling is probably due to the appearance of white spots, the color of the restoration not matching the tooth, and warnings against same-day finishing. But clinicians who have gotten over this initial discomfort insist that the cement is a convenient material. What are the points of divergence in these opinions?

1) Grasping the material's adaptability.
2) Knowing the properties of the material.
3) Following procedures.

In Europe and America, glass ionomer cement was first used by clinicians who feared postoperative pain associated with composite resins. These clinicians had expectations for glass ionomer cement as a restorative material which was safe for pulpal tissue, and they developed techniques to eliminate the undesirable symptoms such as white spots. They searched and strove for favorable results. While the color of composite resins is superior, and therefore attracts clinicians, the attitude that postoperative pain, even if very slight, is intolerable—for both the patient and clinician—is probably the main factor behind clinicians' coming to understand and master the use of glass ionomer cement.

In Japan, the biggest factor behind the dislike for glass ionomer cement is that the procedures required do not match the clinicians' usual procedures. First amalgam, then composite resins, were used for restorative procedures, and so glass ionomer cement was placed using the same handling and procedures. With amalgams and composites, any discomfort, dislodgement, discoloration, or fracture happens several months down the road, so any inadequacy in procedure or material isn't immediately obvious. The success or failure of glass ionomer restorations, however, is clear within ten days. Restorative materials which show failure so clearly are indeed unusual.

(Sueo Saito)

Factors Causing Poor Results for Glass Ionomer Cement Restorations

	Factor	Result
1. Tooth	Decalcified dentin	Loss of restoration, fracture
		Pulpal symptoms
	Exposure	Loss of restoration
	Moisture contamination	
2. Preparation of Materials	Powder<liquid	Long water-sensitive period → water damage
	Air bubbles	Poor appearance, fracture
3. Filling Techniques	More than 1 tooth	Poor contours → air bubbles + poor adhesion
	Finishing too early	More chance of sensitivity H$_2$O of water damage
	Varnish applied	• Too early → poor anatomy
		• Too late → more chance H$_2$O sensitivity when dried
		• Forget drying (no film formed) → water sensitivity
	Syringe not used	Large bubbles → fracture
	Inappropriate same-day finishing	Craze lines, signs of water sensitivity
4. Environment after filling	Cavity form	Many areas unsupported by tooth structure
	Areas of strong forces	Fracture

CHAPTER V

APPLICATIONS FOR GLASS IONOMER CEMENT

APPLICATIONS FOR GLASS IONOMER CEMENT

Section 1: Luting Cement For Inlays and Crowns

Tsugio Iwamoto
Department of Restorative Dentistry
Kanagawa Dental College

Glass ionomer cement was developed in 1972 by A.D. Kent and B.E. Wilson as an esthetic restorative material to replace silicate cement. Research continued on glass ionomers because of their bonding to tooth structure, the positive response of pulpal tissues, and the cement's various other properties which could be incorporated clinically. Through such research, a luting cement for cast restorations was developed, and *Fuji Ionomer Type I* by the GC Corp. was the first such product marketed in Japan.

This early product, however, was not always satisfactory as a luting cement. There were problems with handling, solubility, and especially with film thickness, so clinicians felt that the material was unsuitable as a luting cement. Since then, the manufacturer has improved the product in several areas so that at present, it has properties which rival other luting cements. In short, the clinical evaluation of this cement continues to improve, albeit gradually.

Several required properties can be given for luting cement, and below I would like to mention how well this material satisfies those requirements, and also how the material should be handled clinically in order to meet those requirements.

Handling

The handling of the early products was easily affected by changes in the powder-to-liquid ratio, and because the setting time was short, some difficulties with mixing and handling also occurred. In the more recent products, however, these points have been improved, so that few clinical problems with handling remain. Since the working time is somewhat short, mixing must be completed quickly: in about 40 seconds for small restorations, and in 60 seconds or less for large restorations. The effect of different powder-to-liquid ratios on the cement's properties after setting is not as great as it is on zinc phosphate cement, but use of a standard consistency, if possible, is desirable, and the basic yardstick for this is use of the attached measuring instruments to dispense the powder.

Physical strength

Interlocking forces, which are essential for retaining cast restorations, are greatly affected by the physical strength of the luting material. The strength of compression for glass ionomer cement rivals that of zinc oxide cement, and the tensile strength has a value between that of zinc oxide cement and carboxylic cement, so the cement's properties are appropriate for a luting agent. Since the mechanical strength of the cement is controlled by the powder-to-liquid ratio at the time of mixing, as much powder should be added as possible, but one must be careful to avoid lifting off the restoration because of increased film thickness.

Solubility

The solubility of this material is greater than that of other types of luting cement, and this is a disadvantage. Nevertheless, if the restoration's marginal seal is good, the cement will not directly contact oral fluids when used as a luting cement. Consequently, the margins of the restoration are burnished all around with a burnisher before the cement sets. Care must be taken to prevent or minimize exposure of this cement to the oral environment (Fig. 5-9).

The same considerations also apply to the material's water sensitivity, another disadvantage related to solubility. When seating is completed, varnish is applied to the margin (Fig. 5-10). Water sensitivity must be avoided immediately after the cement sets.

Film Thickness

Proper film thickness is essential for luting cement so that the cast restoration can be seated accurately onto the prepared tooth without the restoration rising up. Recent products show film thickness values which almost satisfy the established standard of less the 30μm. However, because film thickness is greatly influenced by powder-to-liquid ratio at the time of mixing, it is necessary to dispense the powder and liquid as accurately as possible, as stated previously.

Bonding

Bonding to tooth structure is this material's most advantageous feature as a luting agent. A bond strength of about 20 kg/cm² can be obtained between human dentin and the metal alloy about one week after luting, and it is reported that the value drops to about $\frac{1}{5}$ in 60 days. Therefore, rather than relying only on chemical bonding to tooth structure to maintain restorations, we should rely on mechanical interlocking forces obtained from the strength of the cement itself, just as for zinc oxide cement. Therefore, when preparing the tooth, it is essential to provide adequate retention form in the preparation of the tooth cavity and abutment tooth.

Pulpal Irritation

Glass ionomer cement powder uses an organic acid with a normal pH of 5, and this acidity remains for an extended period after setting. According to the results of various biological experiments, however, pulpal irritation is about the same as for carboxylic acid, but less than that of zinc oxide cement. Therefore, this cement can probably be used more safely than the other cement when the preparation in a vital tooth approaches the pulp.

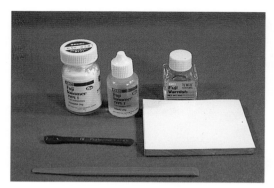

Fig. 5-1. *Fuji Ionomer Type I.* Powder, liquid, mixing pad, varnish, and measuring spoon.

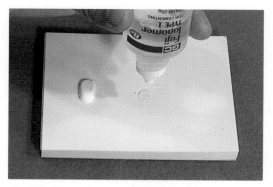

Fig. 5-2. Dispensing powder and liquid.

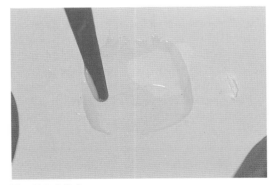

Fig. 5-3. Mixing

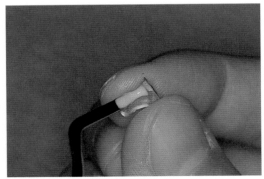

Fig. 5-4. The cement is applied uniformly to the internal surface of the restoration.

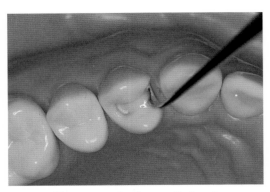

Fig. 5-5. The cement is also applied to the cavity walls.

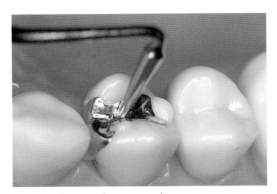

Fig. 5-6. Seating the restoration.

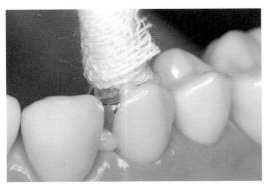

Fig. 5-7. The expressed cement is removed with a cotton pellet or gauze.

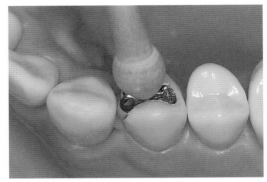

Fig. 5-8. Seating the inlay using a wooden stick.

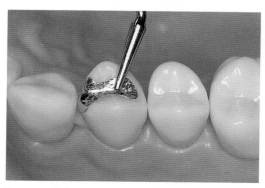

Fig. 5-9. Adequate pressure is applied to the margin of the restoration with a burnisher.

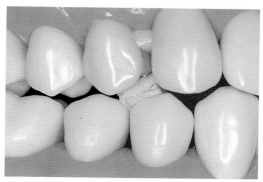

Fig. 5-10. The patient bites down on an orange-wood stick.

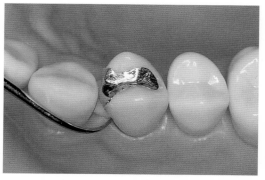

Fig. 5-11. The interproximal surface of the cervical region is carefully examined and the excess cement is removed.

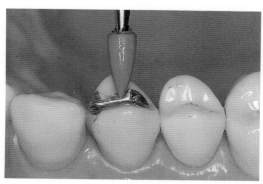

Fig. 5-12. Polishing of the margins with an abrasive point.

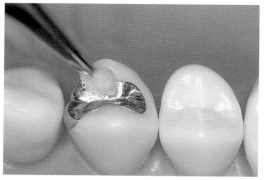

Fig. 5-13. The accompanying varnish is applied to the margins.

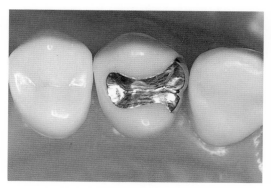

Fig. 5-14. Final polishing of the margins is done with a silicone point.

Section 2: Use As A Restorative Material

A. Esthetic Restoration of Class 3 and 5 Anterior Cavities

Shigeru Katsuyama
Department of Restorative Dentistry
Nihon Dental College

The advantages of glass ionomer cement over composite resins as an esthetic restorative material are the reduced irritation of the pulpal tissue and the simple restorative procedure. However, the drawback is that the presently marketed glass ionomer cement only comes in four shades, so it is difficult to match the shade of the restoration to that of the natural tooth.

Research in this department on 12 products from 3 companies found that 9 products corresponding to the shade guide had $\triangle E > 3$ or greater, confirming that differences in color could indeed be a problem. Further, the brightness of the glass ionomer cement tends to decrease after mixing, starting at 2 minutes 30 seconds and continuing until about 15 minutes (after mixing), then the brightness tends to increase over the next 24 hours. Furthermore, it is clear that the color change at the time of setting is mostly due to a change in the value of the color (Figs. 5-15 through 5-19).

Furthermore, even with the naked eye, it is clear that each product has a different shade guide. It can be concluded from the above that, because the colors of the restorative materials at present and their shade guides are often not consistent, it is necessary—to a certain extent—to practice using the colors. An increase in the number of shade guides and types of shades available would also be desirable.

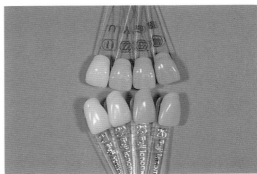

Fig. 5-15. Shade guides.
The shades differ between the commercial products.

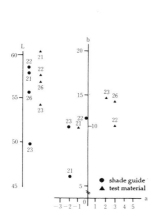

Fig. 5-16. The L value and a-b coordinates of *Fuji Ionomer Type II.*

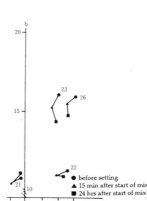

Fig. 5-17. Changes in the a-b values of *Fuji Ionomer Type II.*

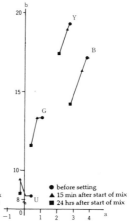

Fig. 5-18. Changes in the a-b values of *Fuji Ionomer Type II.*

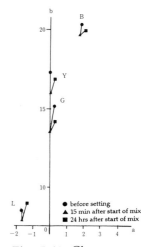

Fig. 5-19. Changes in the a-b values of *Chelon-Fil.*

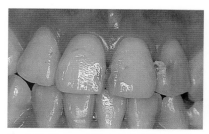

Fig. 5-20. 21-year-old female. Labial of maxillary right and left central incisors and left lateral incisor. Secondary caries can be seen around the restorations.

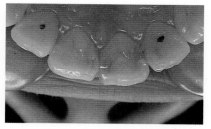

Fig. 5-21. Same case. Lingual of the right and left central incisors and the left lateral incisor. The presence of caries can also be clearly recognized on the lingual.

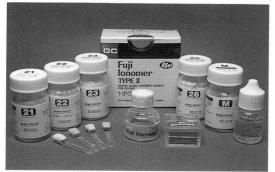

Fig. 5-22. Restorative glass ionomer cement.

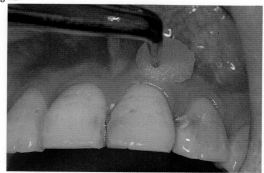

Fig. 5-23. Topical anesthetic is applied to the area where the needle will penetrate.

Class 3 Cavities

The case shown in the accompanying photos is that of a 21-year-old female. Several years before this examination, composite resins were placed on the maxillary central incisors and left lateral incisor. The woman came to the clinic complaining that the margins of the restoration had recently become a little dark, and that there was some sensitivity to cold water (Figs. 5-20, 5-21).

She was diagnosed as having secondary caries around the margins, and it was thought that the caries were quite deep; radiographic diagnosis showed that the caries were in fact quite close to the dental pulp. Evaluation with an electric pulp tester indicated that the tooth was vital.

The tooth was treated by removing the restoration under local anesthetic, placing calcium hydroxide as in an indirect pulp cap in the area closest to the pulp, and restoring it with glass ionomer cement (Fig. 5-22).

After cleansing the tooth, topical anesthetic was applied on the mucosa in the region where the needle would penetrate, and local anesthetic was then administered (Figs. 5-23, 5-24).

The restoration was removed with a high-speed drill using water spray, and a large quantity of soft dentin was found (Fig. 5-25). A spoon excavator was then used to gently remove the soft dentin, and a small round bur was used at slow speed to complete the removal of soft dentin (Fig. 5-26).

The tooth was then isolated with a rubber dam, and a calcium hydroxide pulp cap was placed in the deep section and allowed to set. The cavity was filled using prepared *Fuji Ionomer Type II*, No. 21, starting in the corners of the cavity so that there would be no voids. Pressure was then applied for about 5 minutes using a celluloid strip. After checking the hardness, varnish was applied and the patient was sent home after waiting for the initial set.

She returned to the clinic 3 days later, and confirmed upon questioning that she was not aware of any symptoms. Finishing procedures were carried out after checking to see that there were no problems with the

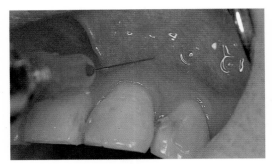

Fig. 5-24. Local anesthetic for the patient.

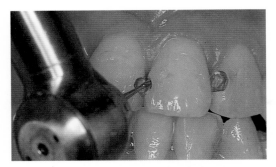

Fig. 5-25. A large quantity of soft dentin was found.

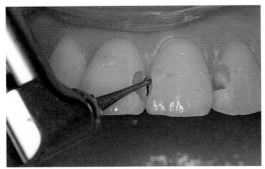

Fig. 5-26. Cavity after removal of soft dentin.

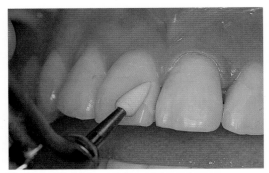

Fig. 5-27. Finishing with a white point.

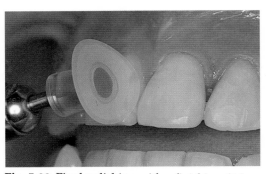

Fig. 5-28. Final polishing with a finishing disk.

restoration, including overhangs, and the contact area of the restoration and the tooth surface was finished using a white stone point under a stream of water (Fig. 5-27).

Next, the interproximal surfaces were finished using polishing strips, and finally, polishing disks were used under a stream of water to complete the finishing (Figs. 5-28, 5-29).

Example of a Class 5 Cavity

This 59-year-old male presented with the chief complaint of sensitivity to cold water on his maxillary right second premolar. His oral hygiene was favorable and gingiva

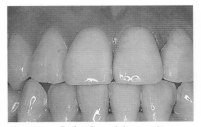

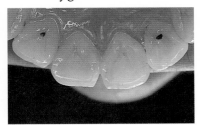

Fig. 5-29. Labial and lingual view of the right and left central incisors and the left lateral incisor after restoration.

104

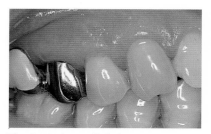

Fig. 5-30. A small defect was seen in the cervical region of the maxillary right first premolar.

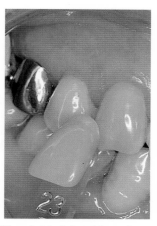

Fig. 5-31. Matching the shade.

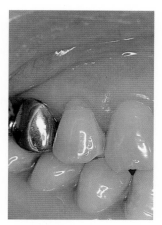

Fig. 5-32. Cavity preparation completed.

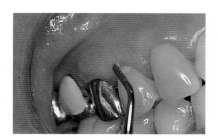

Fig. 5-33. Placing the restorative material.

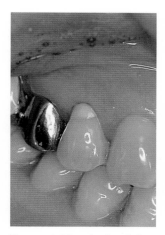

Fig. 5-34. The shade of the restoration is too white.

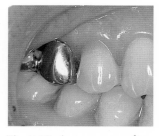

Fig. 5-35. Appearance after the restoration was redone.

were normal. There was a shallow lesion in the cervical region of the maxillary first premolar, and slight pain occurred when the lesion was scratched (Fig. 5-30). We then went directly to choosing a matching shade from the shade guide and restored the tooth with No. 26 (Fig. 5-31).

The surface layer of the lesion was removed using a small round bur, and the gingival wall was made a little deeper. Cement was mixed using the recommended powder-to-liquid ratio, and this was placed with a spatula-type instrument for filling.

Care was taken so that there was no excessive overhang, especially at the gingival cavity margin (Fig. 5-33).

After about 5 minutes, the start of the set was verified, and varnish was applied with a cotton pellet. Then, after allowing for the completion of the initial set of the cement, the patient was sent home.

One week later he returned to the clinic. The shade of the restoration was a little too white, so it was removed (Fig. 5-34) and restored again (Fig. 5-35). No subsequent problems were encountered.

B. Restoration of Cervical Abrasion Lesions

Hideo Onose
Department of Restorative Dentistry
Nippon University School of Dentistry

Cervical abrasion lesions are difficult to treat. Patients with these lesions usually have a loss of hard tissue due to abrasion, mostly from brushing. These lesions usually appear on the labial and buccal surfaces of the cervical region of several teeth in a row, and hypersensitivity on the surface often arises with the lesions.

The first symptom of these patients is the loss of some enamel on the cervical region of the tooth, but since initially there is no pain, most patients do not sense a problem. If at this point, however, the root is exposed, it is more easily abraded than enamel. When the abrasion reaches the dentin, dentinal tubules are either closed by making the dentin finer or new hard tissue is added to the appropriate wall of the pulp chamber; it depends on the speed of the abrasion. If the defensive reactions of the affected tooth are not good enough, however, symptoms of hypersensitivity may arise.

Hypersensitivity arising from a cervical abrasion lesion is not related to its size or depth, but rather, deep lesions in which it appears that the pulp is almost exposed have virtually no sensitivity, and in contrast, hypersensitivity often occurs in really shallow lesions or when the lesion can hardly be detected. Applying glass ionomer cement has recently been proposed as a method of treating the cases of hypersensitivity in lesions which are essentially undetectable, and cervical cement has been marketed for such an application (Figs. 5-54 through 5-57).

Whether these lesions should be restored is still debatable, as the restorations have a high frequency of being lost, but since restorative materials with superior adhesion to tooth structure have been developed, there have been fewer cases of lost restorations. Also, experience shows that the hypersensitivity decreases when the lesion is restored with a material which has a seal like glass ionomer cement.

There are certain points which need particular attention when restoring these lesions with glass ionomer cement. One is to produce the greatest adhesion of tooth structure to cement possible, and the other, a disadvantage of this cement, is to make the white spot on the surface from water sensitivity as small as possible, thus improving esthetics.

In accordance with the theory of adhesion, cleansing of the surface of the lesion is important for adhesion to the tooth structure. The tooth surface of the lesion seems to be smooth to the naked eye, but in fact, it is covered with calculus-type deposits. The dentist can use dentin conditioner, an aqueous solution of 1% polyacrylic acid, for cleansing. If this conditioner is used for 20 - 30 seconds and the cement restoration placed immediately after rinsing and drying, the cement's adhesive properties can be increased.

It is necessary to keep the cement away from moisture from the start of mixing until the cement is set, thus preventing water sensitivity. This means that the cement must be handled very quickly in the clinic, and must also be carried so that it does not contact moisture. A syringe is used so that the transport of the cement paste and filling of the cavity can be accomplished in one step. Also, a matrix fit to the size of the cavity is adjusted and set aside before the operation and is used until the cement sets so that moisture contamination is avoided as much as possible. Pressure is applied, if possible, for over 10 minutes, and then the matrix is removed and varnish be applied. The following clinical case will illustrate the proper restorative techniques.

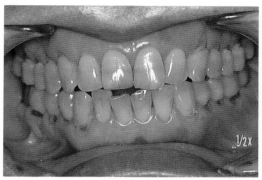

Fig. 5-36. Typical case of cervical abrasion lesions.

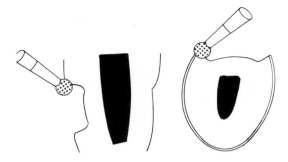

Fig. 5-37. Treatment of the cavity margin. It is designed so that the glass ionomer cement cavity margin is as thick as possible. A groove is therefore provided.

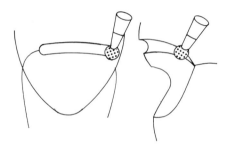

Fig. 5-38. Circumferential groove of the cavity margin. A circumferential groove is made in the cavity margin to prevent marginal fracture of the glass ionomer cement.

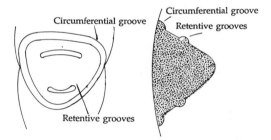

Fig. 5-39. Retentive grooves in the cavity wall. These prevent loss of the glass ionomer cement after it sets, and also serve as a starting point for filling.

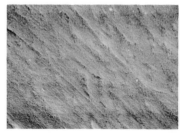
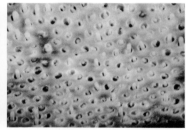
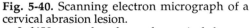

Fig. 5-40. Scanning electron micrograph of a cervical abrasion lesion.
Left: Untreated surfaces of a cervical abrasion lesion.
Right: Surface of a cervical abrasion lesion after 20 second treatment with dentin conditioner (x2000).

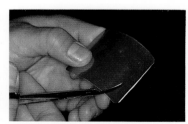

Fig. 5-41. Custom made matrix using an aluminum can.

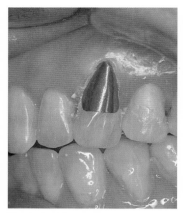

Fig. 5-42. Matrix try-in.

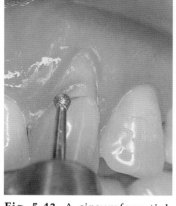

Fig. 5-43. A circumferential groove is made with a round bur.

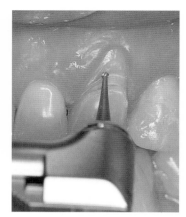

Fig. 5-44. Providing retentive grooves with a round bur.

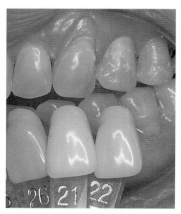

Fig. 5-45. Selecting the shade.

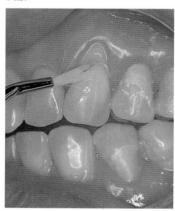

Fig. 5-46. Cleansing the surface with dentin conditioner.

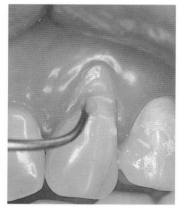

Fig. 5-47. Filling the retentive grooves. A syringe is used for the bulk of the material, but since air bubbles form easily in the groove, the air bubbles are removed with an explorer.

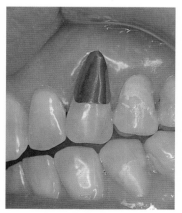

Fig. 5-48. Applying pressure with a matrix.

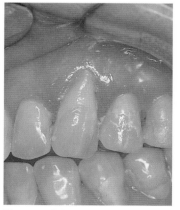

Fig. 5-49. Matrix removed.

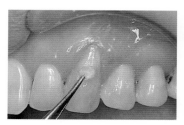

Fig. 5-50. Applying varnish.

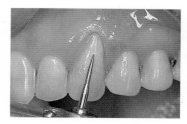

Fig. 5-51. Contouring anatomy with a pointed diamond finishing bur.

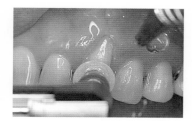

Fig. 5-52. Polishing.

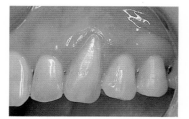

Fig. 5-53. Completed glass ionomer restoration.

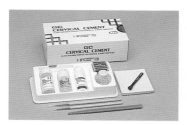

Fig. 5-54. cervical cement.

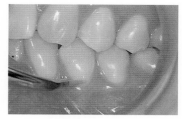

Fig. 5-55. Applying cervical cement. It is painted on thinly with a delicate touch.

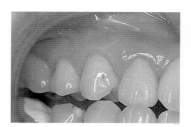

Fig. 5-56 a. Cervical cement applied to the maxillary right first premolar. The cement is barely visible to the naked eye.

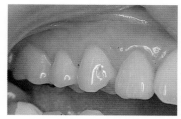

Fig. 5-56 b. One month after placement.

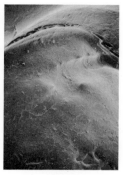

Fig. 5-57. Surface coated with cervical cement (scanning electron micrograph). By applying the cervical cement, the rough spots are soon worn off, and the surface becomes smooth.

C. Restoration of Root Caries

Hideo Onose
Department of Restorative Dentistry
Nippon University Dental School

Glass ionomer cement is one of the few restorative materials which is appropriate for root caries. That is, because of the location of these caries in the root surface, the choice of materials for treatment is quite limited. The cavity is usually near the dental pulp, and in regions where it is difficult to provide retention form in the surrounding existing tooth structure, where there is no healthy enamel surrounding the lesion, and where esthetics are sometimes demanded.

Consequently, an appropriate material is one such as this cement, which bonds to tooth structure, does not have harmful effects on living tissues such as the pulp, has esthetic qualities, and sacrifices little healthy tooth.

These lesions have a shallow nature and follow the line of the necks of the teeth, and often have progressed to a large extent. Periodontal disease is a related disease, and the exposure of root surface by periodontal disease becomes a precondition of this disease. Therefore, there are several points which must be paid attention to when treating these patients.

The first is to prioritize the treatment of the periodontal patient. Removal of calculus, and if necessary, thorough scaling of the root surface is carried out; plaque control by the patient is strictly enforced, and the periodontal disease is brought under control. In particular, the inflammation and swelling of the gingival tissues should be decreased. Once the entire lesion can be seen, treatment of the root caries and removal of carious tissue becomes easy, without any concern over hemorrhaging from the periodontal tissues. If the patient complains about pain (such as hypersensitivity) at this time, as much of the softened carious tissue is removed as possible with a spoon excavator or a round bur, and the entire lesion is sealed with a material which adheres to dental tissues (such as carboxylate cement), so plaque control such as brushing can be carried out painlessly.

There are additional points which need attention for placing restorations with glass ionomer cement. The reasons for using this cement for root caries is, as in the cases of abrasion lesions outlined in the previous section, that it bonds to tooth structure and has good esthetics. Therefore, it is necessary to consider cleansing the surface of the cavity covered with the smear layer for bonding to tooth structure. *G.C. Dentin Conditioner*, an aqueous solution of 10% polyacrylic acid, has been developed to remove this from the surface of the cavity.

However, it has been reported that when glass ionomer cement is used, the acidity of the cement paste has the same effect of removing the smear layer, and that bond strength does not decline. Therefore, the cement paste is placed as quickly as possible after rinsing the cavity surface with water and drying, without using conditioner. At this time, if saliva, periodontal exudate, or blood flows into the cavity, the bond strength of the cement decreases dramatically. Isolation should be considered when placing this cement, and effective use of a syringe and matrix are important clinical operations to prevent water sensitivity of the surface, as was discussed in the previous section.

Below, the restorative techniques will be illustrated with a clinical example.

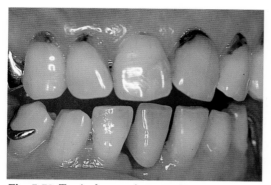

Fig. 5-58. Typical case of root caries.

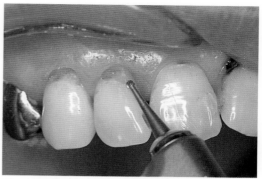

Fig. 5-59. Removal of caries with a round bur.

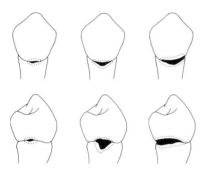

Fig. 5-60. Established outline form. The outline form is not especially extended into self-cleansing areas. It is a smooth, curved outline.

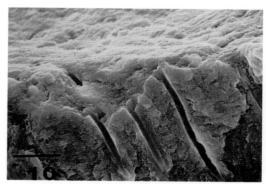

Fig. 5-61. Smear layer on dentin (scanning electron micrograph).

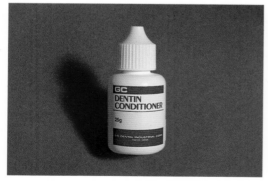

Fig. 5-62. *G.C. Dentin Conditioner*. 10% poly-acrylic acid is the main ingredient.

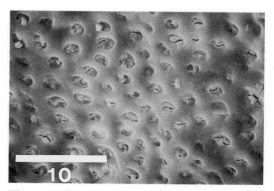

Fig. 5-63. Dentin surface after treating with dentin conditioner for 20 seconds. Dentin plugs can be seen in the dentinal tubules.

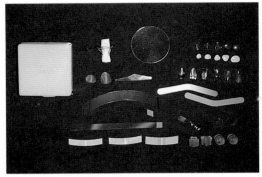

Fig. 5-64. Various matrixes.

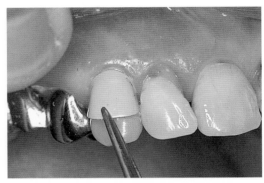

Fig. 5-65. Trying in the matrix for the cavity.

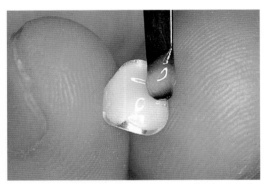

Fig. 5-66. Applying the cement to the internal surface of the matrix. The air bubbles on the surface disappear.

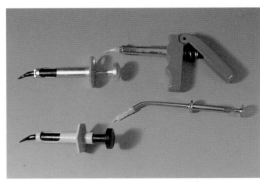

Fig. 5-67. Various filling syringes. These can be used for composite resins.

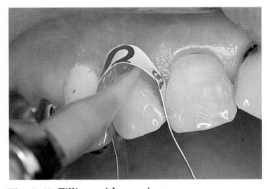

Fig. 5-68. Filling with a syringe.

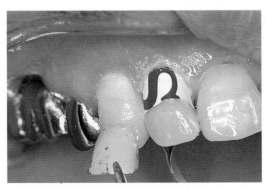

Fig. 5-69. Pressure applied using the matrixes.

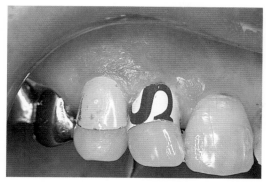

Fig. 5-70. Pressure applied using the matrixes. Ready-made, custom made matrixes.

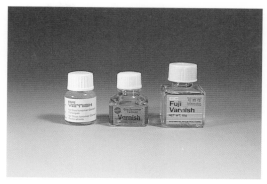

Fig. 5-71. Varnishes.

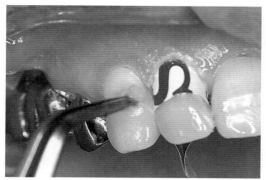

Fig. 5-72. Applying varnish.

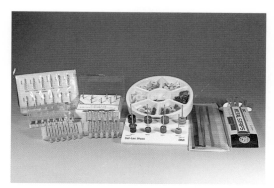

Fig. 5-73. Finishing materials.

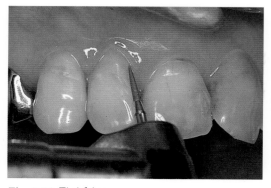

Fig. 5-74. Finishing.

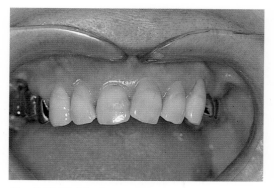

Fig. 5-75. Finished restorations.

Section 3: Glass Ionomer Cement In Pedodontics

Ikuo Omori
Tsurumi University School of Dentistry
Pedodontics Department

The Development of Pit and Fissure Sealants

The use of pit-and-fissure sealants to prevent pit-and-fissure caries was reported by Takeuchi et al[L1] in Japan in 1966, and by Buonocore et al[L2] in the United States at about the same time. That was the beginning.

The main components of the sealants used in that research were cyanoacrylate monomer and methyl methacrylate polymer. *Nuva Seal*[L3] was then developed in 1970: it used a mixture of Bis-GMA and methyl methacrylate monomer as its main component, and was cured by exposure to long wavelength (366 nm) ultraviolet light for 20 to 30 seconds.

Nuva Seal is no longer used because of the possible harmful effects to living tissues such as skin from exposure to the long wavelengths of ultraviolet light that the cement required to set.

In the 1970s, chemically polymerizing types of sealants catalyzed by various chemical substances were developed,[L6] and became widely used clinically.

At present, the main component of the most popular chemically cured sealants is dimethacrylate. Bis-GMA is the main component of the monomer, and a BPO-amino type catalyst is used for polymerization.

In addition to these chemically cured sealants, light-cured sealants which polymerize and harden by exposure to certain visible light have recently been developed and are now used clinically.[L26] Even though these sealants use visible light (wavelength

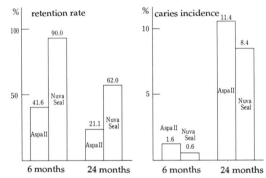

Fig. 5-76. Sealant retention rate and caries incidence for glass ionomer cement (*ASPA II*) and resin sealant (*Nuva Seal*). (Williams, B and Winter, G.B., 1976)

= 400-700 nm), the effective wavelengths for polymerization are actually in the 400-490nm range. Since the sealants are polymerized and set by this blue light, their usage spread quickly, following the spread of light-cured composite resins.

Glass ionomer cement was discovered by Wilson[A2], and it was developed as a dental cement which sets by the reaction of aluminosilicate and either polyacrylic acid or a copolymer of acrylic and itaconic acids.

Three types of glass ionomer cement were developed by GC Corp.: luting cement (*Type I*, 1977), restorative (*Type II*, 1977), and sealant (*Type III*, 1985). The fact that materials for different purposes were developed from one cement is common knowledge.

At that time, research on additives affecting the setting process of glass ionomer cement progressed, and it became clear that the addition of a small quantity of (+)tartaric acid was effective, and at present, (+)tartaric

114

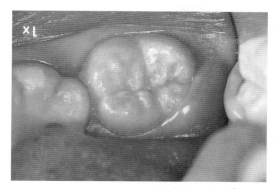

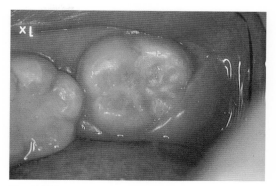

Fig. 5-77 a. 12 year, 2-month-old female. Glass ionomer cement restoration on left mandibular second molar. **a:** before restoration **b:** after restoration

Fig. 5-77 b.

acid is added to all glass ionomer cement.[C70]

The physical properties of the glass ionomer cement developed in 1971 were markedly improved over the next ten or more years, as stated above. Because the presence of water during the setting process strongly affects the physical properties of glass ionomer cement, an adequately dry environment must be maintained from the start of mixing, through the completion of the placement or filling, and until set. By improving the setting process, the time period in which one has to be careful of water sensitivity has been reduced, and we now have the advantage of a longer working time in the clinic.

This improved handling is an especially large advancement for Type III (glass ionomer sealant), which is used mostly for children.

Glass Ionomer Sealant

Williams et al[L7], used *ASPA II* glass ionomer cement as a sealant and compared its retention rates in pits and fissures and the incidence of pit-and-fissure caries with that of *Nuva-Seal*, which was widely used at that time, and with other chemically cured sealants. As shown in Figure 5-76, the reports found that 2 years after sealing the pit and fis-

sures, *Nuva-Seal* had a retention rate of 62%, while *ASPA II* had a retention rate of 21.1%, so most of the cement sealants were lost.

The incidence of caries for the sealed teeth was 8.4% with *Nuva Seal*, and even with *ASPA II*, it was not more then 11.4%. When glass ionomer cement is used as a sealant, the retention rate is low compared to resin sealants, but it must be pointed out that there is not a large difference in the incidence of caries. It is thought that the fluoride which makes up approximately 16% of the glass ionomer sealants has an anticariogenic effect. It must be noted that the enamel for the *ASPA II* was also etched for 60 seconds with 50% phosphoric acid in this research.

An additional advantage of glass ionomer sealant is that adhesion to the tooth structure can be expected without acid etching, and as shown in Figure 5-77, it can be applied to the pits and fissures of the occlusal surface of an incompletely erupted tooth for which rubber dam isolation is difficult.

In these types of cases, it is difficult for the tips of the toothbrush bristles to reach into the fissures, and furthermore, because there is no mechanical cleansing from mastication, such areas have an especially high caries susceptibility. When these factors are considered, the application of glass ionomer sealants to this type of incompletely erupted tooth is highly significant. This is also pointed out by the clinical results[L21] on glass ionomer sealants published by G.C. Circle.

Four cases of glass ionomer sealants are shown. Each was an incompletely erupted tooth, and it can be said that these cases of application brought out the strong points of glass ionomer sealants (Figs. 5-78 through 5-81).

Table 5-1. Retention rate of glass ionomer sealants at 6 months in first molars [( ) is %] (Koichi Kawakami, 1986).

	good	fair	poor	total
maxillary	7(17.5)	14(35.0)	19(47.5)	40
	21(52.5)			
mandibular	23(45.1)	19(37.3)	9(17.6)	51
	42(82.4)			
total	30(33.0)	33(36.3)	28(30.7)	91
	63(69.3)			

Advantages of Glass Ionomer Sealants

1. Adhesion to tooth structure can be expected even without acid etching.

2. Fluoride contained in the glass ionomer sealant is released and then is taken up by the enamel, increasing the acid resistance of the tooth and producing an anticariogenic effect.

3. It is possible to use them especially effectively for incompletely erupted teeth which are difficult to isolate with rubber dam.

Pointers for Glass Ionomer Sealants

1. Decreasing the powder:liquid ratio during mixing results in greater solubility of the glass ionomer sealant.

2. High fillings end up receiving occlusal forces which cause marginal breakdown and fracture of the sealant itself.

3. It is necessary to pay attention to the water sensitivity of the glass ionomer sealant. Adequate isolation is essential especially in the setting process.

Cases Using Glass Ionomer Sealants

CASE 1

7 year, 1-month-old female, mandibular left first molar. (Case No. 25924)
Isolation technique: simple   Surface cleansing method: prophy brush, explorer   Oral hygiene: good

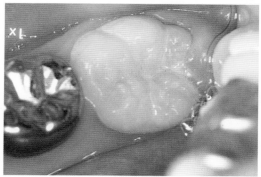 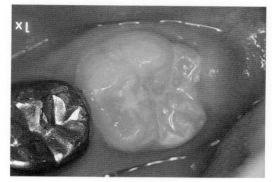

Fig. 5-78 a. Before restoration.   **Fig. 5-78 b.** Immediately after restoration.

region	mesial pit	central pit	distal pit	buccal groove
caries	C_0	C_0	C_1	C_0

CASE 2

6 year, 10-month-old female, maxillary left first molar. (Case No. 26512)
Isolation technique: simple   Surface cleansing method: prophy brush, explorer   Oral hygiene: good

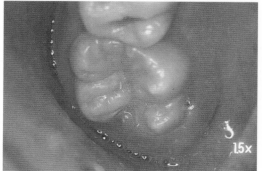 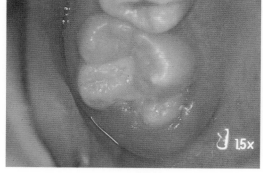

Fig. 5-79 a. Before restoration.   **Fig. 5-79b.** Immediately after restoration.

region	mesial pit	central pit	distal pit	buccal groove	lingual groove
caries	I		I		I

CASE 3
5 year 6 month old female, mandibular right first molar. (Case No. 277985)
    Isolation technique: simple   Surface cleansing method: prophy brush, explorer   Oral hygiene: good

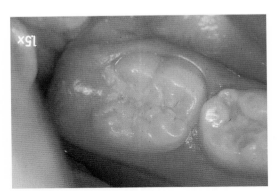

Fig. 5-80 a. Before restoration.

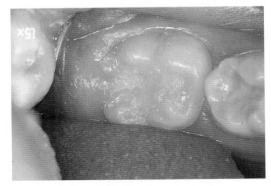

Fig. 5-80 b. Immediately after restoration.

region	mesial pit	central pit	distal pit	buccal groove
caries	C_1	C_1	C_1	C_0

CASE 4
13 year, 1-month-old female, mandibular right second molar. (Case No. 244135)
    Isolation technique: simple   Surface cleansing method: prophy brush, explorer   Oral hygiene: fair

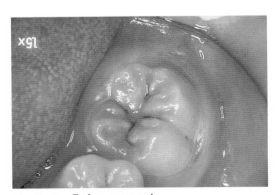

Fig. 5-81 a. Before restoration.

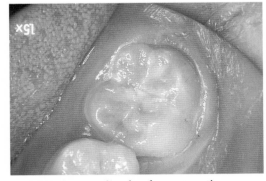

Fig. 5-81 b. Immediately after restoration.

region	mesial pit	central pit	distal pit	buccal groove
caries	C_1	C_1	C_0	C_0

Table 5-2. Number of teeth: 42 (male: 19 teeth, female: 23 teeth).

	first molar	second molar
maxillary	15	7
mandibular	10	10

Table 5-3. Maxillary

tooth	first molar		second molar	
region	M	D	M	D
no. of pits	15	13	7	5

Mandibular

tooth	first molar			second molar		
region	M	C	D	M	C	D
no. of pits	10	10	7	10	10	5

M: mesial pit C: central pit D: distal pit

Table 5-4. Observation period (weeks).

tooth	maxillary		mandibular	
	first molar	second molar	first molar	second molar
longest	9	5	8	8
shortest	3	4	3	3
average	5	4	4	5

Clinical Record of Glass Ionomer Sealants

A total of 42 teeth—first and second molars—which would be difficult to isolate with rubber dam due to their incomplete eruption, were selected as subjects in children who came to the pedodontic clinic at Tsurumi University School of Dentistry. After the occlusal pits and fissures of the teeth were cleansed using a prophy brush and explorer, glass ionomer sealants (*Fuji Ionomer Type III*) were placed, and the retention of the sealant then observed.

The average length of observation was short—only five weeks, but when the clinical results on the retention rate of the original sealants is considered, the observation of the sealant in this short period after placement is also important. Also, since the length of observation was short, no evaluation of incidence of pit-and-fissure caries was carried out.

The number of each type of tooth and the number of pits (for the teeth in the experiment) are shown in Tables 5-2 and 5-3.

The examination of the retention of the glass ionomer sealants was done at the same pedodontics office. The summary of the results are as shown in Tables 5-5 and 5-6. Although the length of observation was dif-

Table 5-5. Retention rate for each pit (retentive pits/total no of pits %).

		M	C	D
maxillary	first molar	12/15 80.0		10/13 76.9
	second molar	6/7 65.7		5/5 100.0
mandibular	first molar	8/10 80.0	8/10 80.0	6/7 85.7
	second molar	7/10 70.0	8/10 80.0	4/5 80.0

Table 5-6. Retention rate for first and second molars (teeth with complete retention/total no of teeth %).

maxillary	first molar	12/15 80.0
	second molar	6/7 65.7
mandibular	first molar	6/10 80.0
	second molar	6/10 80.0

ferent, compared to the results shown previously, the results are almost the same.

A good technique based on these studies might be to protect the pits and fissures with glass ionomer cement when the eruption is still incomplete, and then proceed to resin sealants when eruption is sufficient.

If one considers the high incidence of caries in the first and second molars of children in Japan at present, the frequent occurrence of pit-and-fissure caries during childhood could be prevented, and the development of incipient caries could be arrested by skillfully using glass ionomer sealants and resin sealants. The significance of these prophylactic measures could be very large.

The handling of *Fuji Ionomer Type III* was compared to the resin sealants in a questionnaire to doctors in this department, and it is probably necessary to point out and consider the difficulties in handling the material when placing it on the teeth. Three cases showing results after a relatively long period in the oral cavity are illustrated in Figures 5-82 through 5-84.

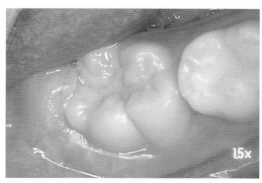

Fig. 5-82. 3 months after placing glass ionomer sealant. Mandibular left first molar: marginal fracture (+), caries (-).

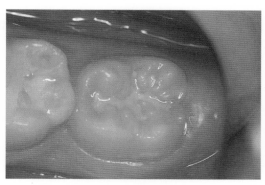

Fig. 5-83. 4 months after placing glass ionomer sealant. Mandibular right second molar: marginal fracture (+), caries (-).

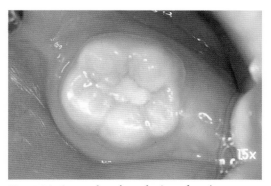

Fig. 5-84. 6 months after placing glass ionomer sealant. Mandibular right first molar sealant fracture (+), marginal fracture (+), caries (-).

Table 5-7. Number of teeth.

	first primary molar	second primary molar
maxillary	3	6
mandibular	1	1

Table 5-8. Observation period (weeks).

longest 12.6	shortest 2	average 9

Table 5-9. Symptoms of discomfort.

region	maxillary first primary molar	maxillary second primary molar	mandibular first primary molar	mandibular second primary molar
loss of crown	0	0	0	0
pain	0	0	0	0

As a Luting Agent

Glass ionomer cement is beginning to be used in place of zinc phosphate cement to lute crowns for primary teeth in the field of pedodontics. The results of using *Fuji Ionomer Type I* for luting prefabricated crowns for primary teeth on first and second molars of young children who came to the pedodontic clinic at Tsurumi University School of Dentistry are as shown in Figures 5-82 through 5-84.

This was an experiment with a small number of cases, 11, but during the average period of observation of nine weeks, there were no cases of lost crowns or symptoms of discomfort.

As a Restorative Material

In seven cases using *Fuji Ionomer Type II* as a lining in primary teeth or young permanent teeth in patients going to the pedodontic clinic at Tsurumi University School of Dentistry, no symptoms of discomfort were seen in a clinical experiment with an average period of observation of 13 weeks. It is thought that restorative glass ionomer cement can be used in the field of pedodontics as a lining and restorative material in a manner similar to that of calcium hydroxide and composite resin.

Furthermore, we believe that the cement is appropriate for sealing cavities and for build-ups after pulpotomies.

Section 4: Glass Ionomer Cement As A Lining Material

Koichi Narikawa, Benji Fujii
Department of Restorative Dentistry
Osaka Dental College

There are two different opinions with regard to the use of composite resins restorations. One is that, in principle, it is necessary to have some kind of procedure to protect the dental pulp, and the other is that if the restoration is done with resin which bonds directly, there is no need for a special procedure.

The debate continues as to which technique should be used, but here I will address the techniques used for cement linings, starting with the much-written-about era of silicate cement and MMA resins, and then continuing on up through the most orthodox method used today, a clinically reliable technique.

The harmful effects of restorative materials for anterior teeth on pulpal tissues have been widely discussed since the development of silicate cement and MMA resins. Much continues to be written about the composite resins of today. The causes of pulpal injury are harmful effects that the restorative material itself possesses, bacteria left in the cavity, and marginal leakage. If a cement lining is used properly, even if it does not go so far as to completely insulate the pulp from all the harmful effects, at least dentists can feel comfortable with their efforts in the clinic.

Zinc phosphate cement was the original cement used for luting, but the cement itself is certainly not something that protects the pulp. Instead, it has a harmful, though temporary, effect on the pulp. This material has become clinically accepted because the duration of the harmful effects is short.

A report has also been published on an experiment on the marginal leakage of MMA resin and composite resin which illustrated that the leakage was stopped splendidly with a layer of cement lining.

However, zinc phosphate cement does not adhere to tooth, especially dentin, and fear of leakage from below the cement lining can be considered. Cement which contains a carboxyl radical in the liquid, i.e., carboxylic acid and glass ionomer cement, adheres to tooth structure and also has a favorable marginal seal. The appearance of this kind of fundamental material as a lining cement was desirable and a company in Japan has already marketed a fine product.

The color resembles that of the crowns of teeth but because it has a different transparency, it is easily distinguished from tooth structure. Even if lining cement sticks out from the cavity accidently during work, differentiation and removal is not a problem.

For composite resin restorations, acid etching of the enamel is a required procedure, and the lining cement is affected more or less by the acid during etching. In general, the clinician moves onto the acid treatment 2 or 3 minutes after placing the cement lining, and since the lining is attacked by acid and water earlier than its setting time, the solubility of the cement becomes an important consideration. In addition, solubility in natural tooth fluids are an important problem.

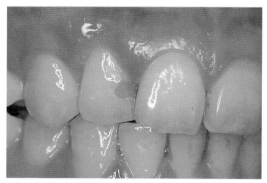

Fig. 5-85. Labial, before treatment, 31-year-old female. A composite resin restoration was placed 7 years prior, and because of the discoloration, she came to the clinic complaining that it was unesthetic.

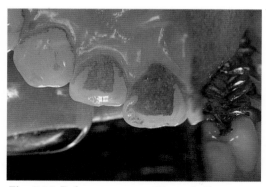

Fig. 5-86. Before treatment. Lingual. She was a smoker and hygiene on the lingual was not good. This probably also affected the composite resin.

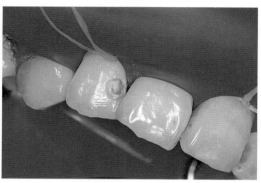

Fig. 5-87. The discolored resin was removed and rubber dam placed. Rubber dam retainers were placed on the first premolars. A ligature was tied around the tooth and retraction of the gingiva was increased.

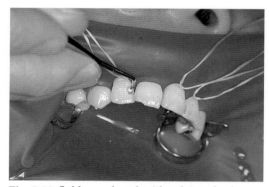

Fig. 5-88. Subbase placed with calcium hydroxide (dycal). (Indirect pulp cap.)

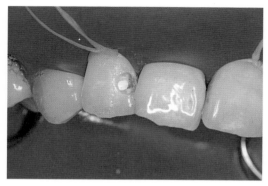

Fig. 5-89. Because of the high solubility of calcium hydroxide in tooth fluids, the area it covers is kept to a minimum. Try not to get any on the cavity wall.

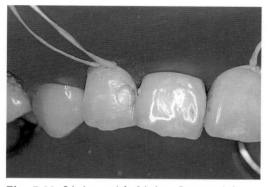

Fig. 5-90. Lining with *Lining Cement* (glass ionomer cement) completed. It is placed so that no exposed dentin remains. The dentinal tubules near the cervical wall are completely sealed, especially in Class 3 restorations.

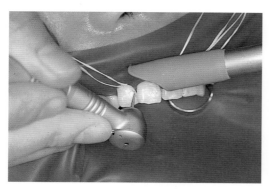

Fig. 5-91. A bevel is provided around the enamel cavity wall with a flame-shaped fine diamond.

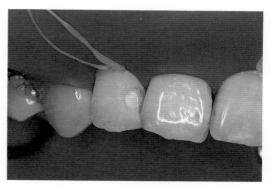

Fig. 5-92. Bevel completed. Even if the lining material stuck to the cavity margin, it can be removed at this point. A bevel about 1 mm wide is appropriate.

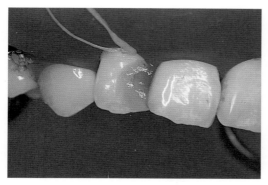

Fig. 5-93. Enamel is etched for 15 to 30 seconds. As much as possible, the etchant is not extended to unneeded areas such as the adjacent teeth or beyond the bevel.

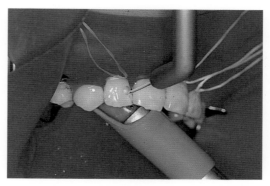

Fig. 5-94. Etchant is rinsed away with water for 15 to 30 seconds. If etchant remains, it hinders polymerization of the composite resin.

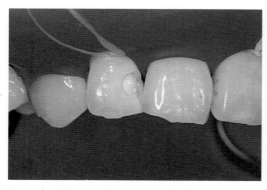

Fig. 5-95. Drying. Rinsing and drying under the rubber dam are extremely easy, with no saliva welling up.

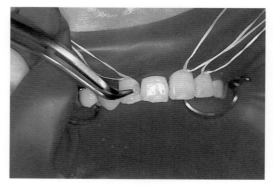

Fig. 5-96. Applying bonding agent with a sponge. It is not rubbed in. The bonding agent is allowed to spread out by itself on the etched surface.

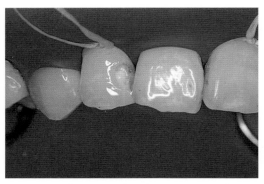

Fig. 5-97. The excess bonding agent is blown away, but in some recent products, it is recommended that the bonding agent be left as a thick layer, so whatever procedure is appropriate for the material should be followed.

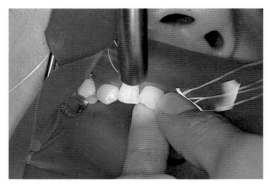

Fig. 5-98. Polymerization of the bonding agent. If the bonding agent touches the adjacent tooth, the teeth will be stuck together, so a matrix strip is introduced between the teeth, and the bonding agent is cured.

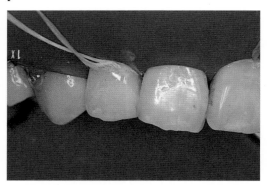

Fig. 5-99. Restoration completed. Since the shade of light cured resins after polymerization becomes more white than the resin paste, it is desirable to make a special shade guide.

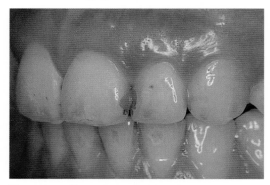

Fig. 5-100. Contralateral side of same patient, before restoration. There are composite resin restorations, but the stain and discoloration are marked.

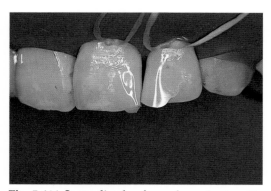

Fig. 5-101. Immediately after polymerization. It is cured after filling with the resin paste and applying pressure.

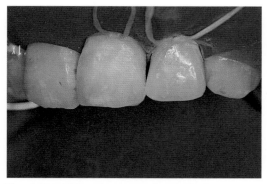

Fig. 5-102. Trimming completed. Rather than finishing on the same day, it is desirable to do it on a later day.

Section 5: Glass Ionomer Cement As A Base
A. Bases For Inlays And Amalgams

Koichi Narikawa, Benji Fujii
Osaka Dental College
Restorative Dentistry Department

Some would say that we have entered the era of using composite resins for restoring molars, and but others would say that metallic restorations are still in the mainstream. The latter view is especially prevalent for molars which bear the burden of heavy occlusal forces.

When restoring large deep caries, it is necessary to replace the lost dentin and have a foundation to support the outer restoration. This foundation is called a base, and it should have properties much like dentin.

For a long time, a hard mix of luting cement was used to achieve this objective, and its use has become a very convenient technique. The powder in zinc phosphate cement was increased so that the cement had a putty-like consistency which did not stick to the fingers. However, since adhesion to tooth structure could not be expected, it was necessary to provide retention form for the base in healthy dentin.

Furthermore, because there was no seal against microleakage, leakage extended into deep portions of the dentin all at once if the marginal seal of the outer restoration was lost, increasing the danger of possible pulpal injury. In order to ameliorate this situation, the appearance of special base materials which bond to dentin, have strength suitable for dentin, and have good handling qualities was desired.

At present, glass ionomer cement for bases is marketed by several companies, all with glass ionomer as their basic component. Each cement's bonding strength with dentin, physical properties, and handling properties are clinically acceptable. The cement's radiopacity has been improved over that of restorative glass ionomer, but it cannot be said to be adequate for products that do not contain either sintered silver or silver alloy.

When using glass ionomer cement for bases, one must wipe out the image of using a dry mix of cement, as has been established with the original cement bases. The standard technique for glass ionomers is to remove the pathologic dentin and place the cement into the cavity, then to prepare the cavity after more than 24 hours have elapsed. No special retention form is needed for the base when placing the base material, and the cement base is left in this form for over 24 hours to improve the cutting qualities.

These cement bases not only support the outer structure as a simple replacement for dentin, but can also be useful as an outer restoration if left in place for less than a year and a half. The cement is very effective over the long term with respect to observing pulpal changes.

This material can also be applied satisfactorily to making core build-ups for complete coverage crowns, as will be discussed later.

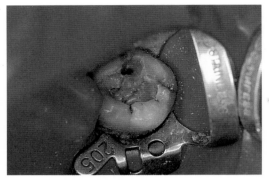

Fig. 5-103. This case had an amalgam restoration which needed to be replaced because of secondary caries. Shown after caries removal. Plan is to prepare a Class 1 cavity.

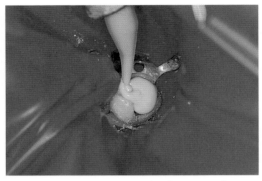

Fig. 5-104. Inserting *Dentin Cement* using a syringe. Increasing the powder to about three times that of the standard makes it easy to use clinically.

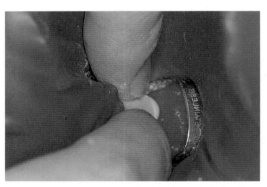

Fig. 5-105. A matrix strip is placed and adequate finger pressure is applied. This is necessary to assure bonding between the *Dentin Cement* and the dentin.

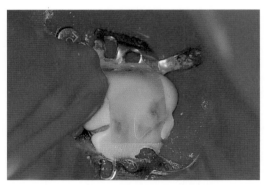

Fig. 5-106. Setting completed. It is desirable to perform the procedures up to this step under a rubber dam.

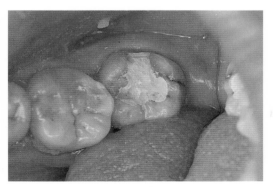

Fig. 5-107. Removal of excess cement. Cement is not left on the cavity margin so that cavity preparation on a later day will be facilitated. The patient is sent home like this for the time being.

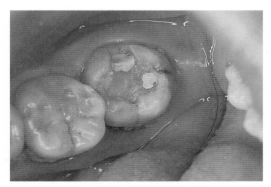

Fig. 5-108. Cavity preparation on a later day is made following the prescribed technique. The base cement cuts with a sensation similar to that of dentin.

CASE 2

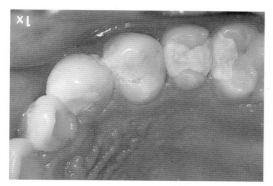

Fig. 5-109. Four months after placing dentin shade *Base Cement*.

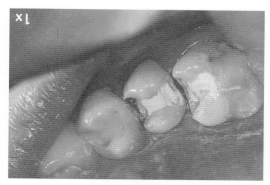

Fig. 5-110. Cavity preparation completed. The axial walls and pulpal floor are formed almost completely by the cement base.

CASE 3

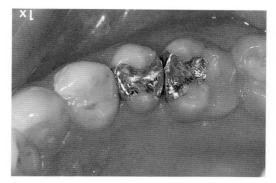

Fig. 5-111. Amalgam restoration. Over one year has passed since restoration, and there is no pain or other signs of discomfort.

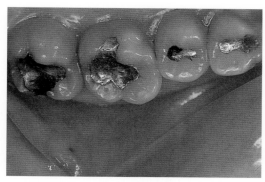

Fig. 5-112. Before treatment. There are caries on the mesial of the maxillary left first premolar and between the first and second molars. The amalgam in the second premolar will simply be replaced.

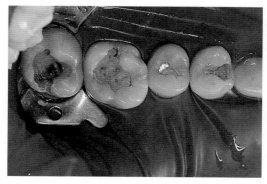

Fig. 5-113. Restorations removed. The caries in the first premolar and the second molar appear quite deep.

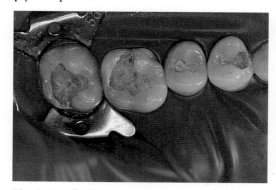

Fig. 5-114. Caries removed. The enamel of the distobuccal cusp of the second molar is unsupported and cuspal coverage is needed. At this point, the design of the cavity should be established.

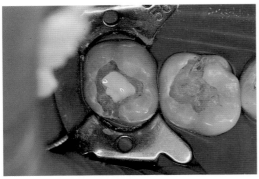

Fig. 5-115. A subbase of calcium hydroxide (dycal) is placed in the deepest area (indirect pulp cap). The caries were chronic and close to the dental pulp, and a subbase is required.

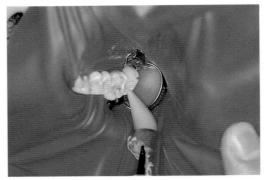

Fig. 5-116. Inserting *Dentin Cement* for bases using a syringe. A matrix band is not used because there is enamel on the interproximal surface.

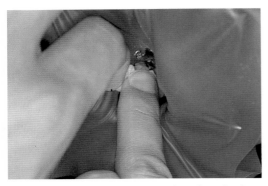

Fig. 5-117. A matrix strip is placed and adequate finger pressure is applied. This is necessary to assure the bonding of the base cement to the dentin.

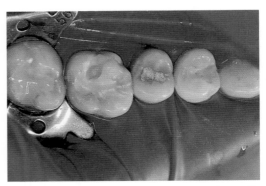

Fig. 5-118. Bases are trimmed. This is done all over with a #6 round bur, and then the small areas are finished with a #2 bur. The patient is sent home like this.

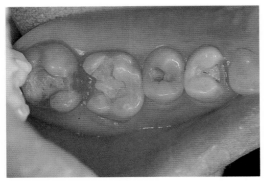

Fig. 5-119. Cavity preparation completed on a later day. The distobuccal cusp of the second molar will be covered as designed in Fig. 5-114.

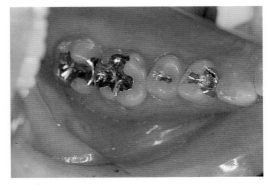

Fig. 5-120. Restorations completed: first premolar MO inlay, second premolar amalgam polished, first molar DOL inlay, and second molar MOB inlay.

CASE 4

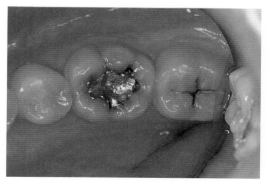

Fig. 5-121. Before treatment. There are extensive caries beneath the inlay on the mandibular first molar extending onto the interproximal surface. The second premolar and the second molar also have caries.

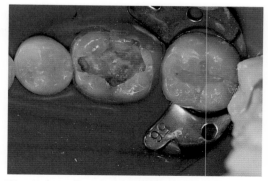

Fig. 5-122. Caries removed from the first molar. Mesial caries have been removed but enamel still remains.

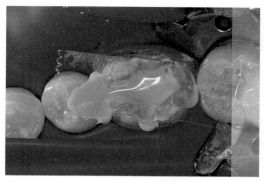

Fig. 5-123. A matrix band is placed between the second premolar and the first molar, and *Dentin Cement* is inserted and pressure applied. After this, the excess cement was trimmed and the patient sent home.

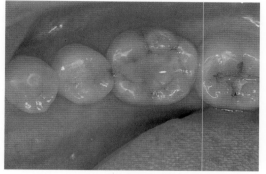

Fig. 5-124. One month later when the patient returned to the clinic. No changes were seen in the temporary cement restoration. The cement was regarded as tooth structure and the cavity was prepared.

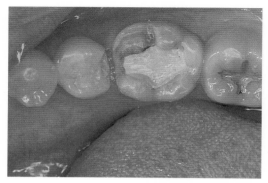

Fig. 5-125. Cavity preparation completed on the second premolar and the first molar. The axial wall of the premolar and the pulpal and axial walls of the molar are almost all formed in cement base.

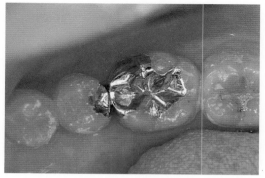

Fig. 5-126. Restorations after insertion. Zinc phosphate cement was used as the luting cement, but glass ionomer cement would have greater adhesion to the cement base.

B. The Sandwich Technique

Koichi Narikawa, Benji Fujii
Department of Restorative Dentistry
Osaka Dental College

When restoring with composite resins, it is necessary to prevent pulpal irritation from microleakage and from the bacteria remaining on the smear layer. On this there is no disagreement, but at present, the debate over techniques to accomplish such goals is confused by various theories. Nevertheless, providing a lining of cement material is the safest technique from the clinician's viewpoint. Leakage seldom reaches pulpal tissue when the cavity is lined with the new carboxylates or glass ionomers, even when the marginal seal appears to be broken, so these materials and their techniques are very useful in the clinic. And needless to say, a base is necessary for composite resin restorations when treating deep caries. These bases can be thought of as similar to bases for inlays and amalgam restorations.

"The sandwich technique" refers to providing a lining or base of glass ionomer cement, then etching both the enamel and cement, and finally placing a composite resin restoration over the cement. Almost all of the dentin in the cavity in this technique is covered by glass ionomer cement. A bond strength of between 30-60 kgf/cm² between the etched glass ionomer cement and the resin is thereby obtained. The sandwich technique is appropriate for: (1) cervical caries, i.e., cases where there is almost no enamel cavity margin in the cervical region, or none can be seen; (2) cases of cervical abrasions; and finally, (3) cases of relatively deep Class 1 and Class 2 caries. Of these, the technique is particularly useful for cases in the cervical region.

When occlusal forces do not need to be borne directly in the cervical region, one can expect to combine both the favorable seal of dentin with glass ionomer and the esthetics and durability of composite resins at the same time. However, when light-cured resin is used, polymerization by light is a short 20-30 seconds. Moreover, due to the tendency of condensation shrinkage to occur toward the layer of filling material, the bonding of the composite resin to the glass ionomer becomes one's enemy, with the glass ionomer separating from the dentin, possibly causing postoperative hypersensitivity. To prevent this kind of phenomenon, the composite resin should be added on top of high-strength glass ionomer cement for bases in the cavity after the glass ionomer cement has set sufficiently, over 24 hours. Also, acid etching is limited to the enamel when filling molars, and the clinician should probably use techniques which do not expect bonding of the glass ionomer cement to the composite resin.

CASE 1

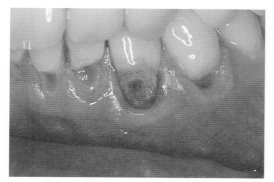

Fig. 5-127. Caries removed. This case started as a cervical abrasion and then became carious, and the patient complained of pain with cold water. The central area is close to the pulp.

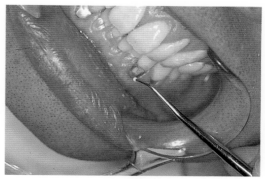

Fig. 5-128. A subbase of calcium hydroxide (dycal) was placed in the deepest area (indirect pulp cap).

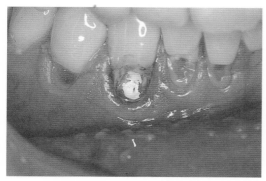

Fig. 5-129. Subbase completed. The subbase is kept as small as possible so that the area of adhesion between the base cement and the dentin is large. In this case, some trimming is required.

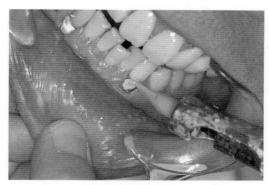

Fig. 5-130. *Dentin Cement* inserted using a syringe.

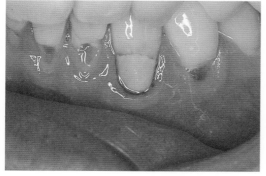

Fig. 5-131. Cement base trimmed. The trimming is done while gently retracting the gingiva with an explorer so that there is no exudate in the area covered by gingiva.

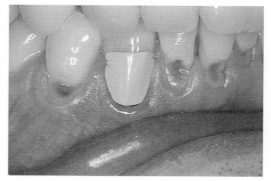

Fig. 5-132. After 2 weeks. There were no symptoms of discomfort when the patient returned to the clinic, and a matrix for the cervical area was tried in.

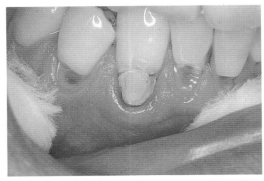

Fig. 5-133. Cavity preparation completed. The incisal enamel is completely exposed, but the other cavity margins are only slightly exposed.

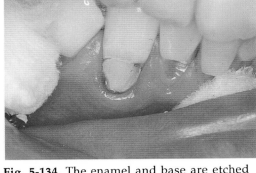

Fig. 5-134. The enamel and base are etched with phosphoric acid, rinsed and dried.

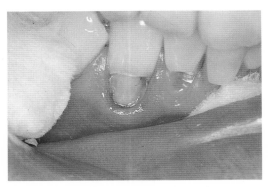

Fig. 5-135. Bonding agent applied. The excess bonding agent is blown away.

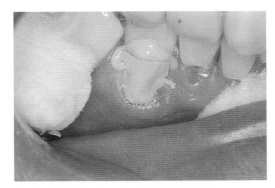

Fig. 5-136. Restored with chemically cured composite resin. Pressure applied with a cervical area matrix.

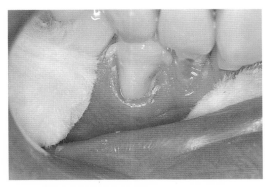

Fig. 5-137. The resin has set. The restoration is completed by finishing on a later day.

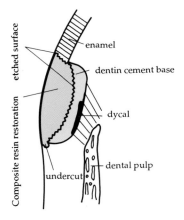

Fig. 5-138. Diagram of the sandwich technique. When there is sufficient enamel, the glass ionomer base is placed up near the cavity margin, and depending on the case, undercuts may be provided.

CASE 2

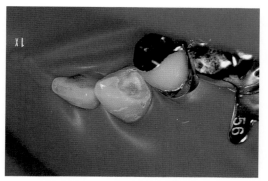

Fig. 5-139. Before restoration. Caries removal completed. Deep caries suspected.

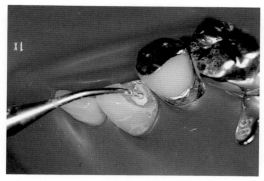

Fig. 5-140. A subbase of calcium hydroxide (dycal) is placed (indirect pulp cap).

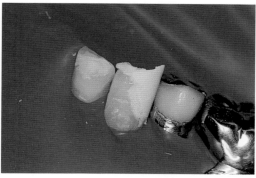

Fig. 5-141. Cement base completed with dentin shade *Base Cement*.

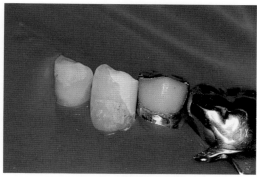

Fig. 5-142. Cement base trimming completed. The patient is sent home at this point, and the tooth is prepared again and restored with composite resin at a later day.

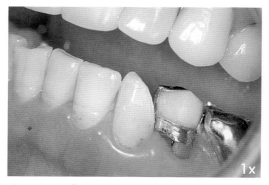

Fig. 5-143. Cement base completed. Etching, rinsing, applying bonding agent, and polymerization are done after this using regular techniques.

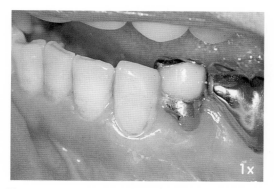

Fig. 5-144. Composite resin restoration completed.

C. Cement Base As A Core Material

Koichi Narikawa, Benji Fujii
Department of Restorative Dentistry
Osaka Dental College

In the sense that both bases and cores fill in for lost dentin, and that they are dentin substitutes which support the coronal restoration, they have very similar properties. However, the differences are that while bases are thought of mostly for vital teeth and have relatively high interior properties, cores are mainly for nonvital teeth and the external properties are relatively high. Nevertheless, both are basically dentin substitutes, and it is possible to use base materials for cores. In vital teeth where caries are extensive and a crown is required, both cores and bases can be thought of at the same time, but if the teeth become nonvital, various conditions must be considered.

First, when physical properties such as the strength, especially compressive strength and elasticity, are considered, cement for bases are superior to the composite resins frequently used for cores in the clinic today. However, the opposite is true of tensile strength and resilience. That is, the hardness of the base is brittle, and the hardness of the composite resins for cores is inferior in terms of tenacious strength. When these differences are considered, it is only natural to conclude that there are a limited number of cases in which base materials can be used for cores.

We think appropriate cases are those in which more than two walls of dentin help bear the occlusal stresses, and the dentin being replaced is relatively interior dentin. Therefore, cases in which only root remains or in which base material covers the crown of a prepared abutment tooth should be avoided as much as possible.

In this type of case, the use of a screw-type post is desired, with the end of the post in the cement base to spread the occlusal forces throughout the base, so the forces do not concentrate at the apical tip of the post, and the danger of root fracture is small. At any rate, bases in vital and nonvital teeth should probably be stopped in a manner similar to MODBL cuspal coverage.

As same fundamental properties are expected of both bases and cores, and it would be convenient to have one material for which all procedures could be completed. The fact is, however, that materials which attempt to represent both have both strong points and shortcomings, and we can not get by with just one material. Many research topics on these types of materials still remain.

At present, it is also necessary to carefully consider using base material for cores in nonvital teeth, and one should not apply one material thoughtlessly for a different use. This is an era of specialty materials, not one of convenience in which a product is used only because its use is possible.

We anxiously await a material which can be used as both a core and a base, without fears, adequately fulfilling both functions.

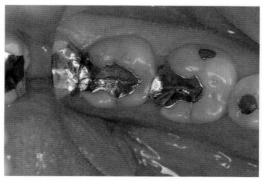

Fig. 5-145. Before restoration. Initial restoration completed one month ago, but pain with cold water and on occluding continued, causing difficulty masticating.

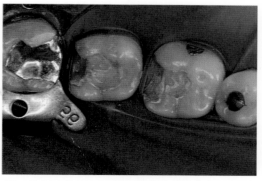

Fig. 5-146. Inlays removed. A thick layer of glass ionomer luting cement still remains.

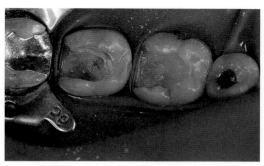

Fig. 5-147. Cement removed. Pulp exposures on pulp horns on distolingual of mandibular rt. first molar and mesiolingual of mandibular rt. second molar. History indicated removal pulp removal.

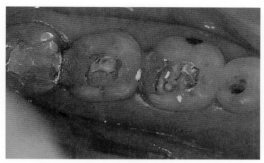

Fig. 5-148. Pulp treatment completed. The pink cement served as the distal wall for the pulpectomy. The outline of the cavity form is designed at this time.

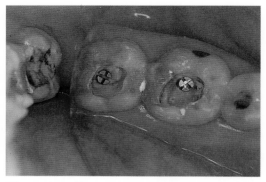

Fig. 5-149. Screw-type posts placed. It is thought that it is fine to use a base-type cement when cementing the posts.

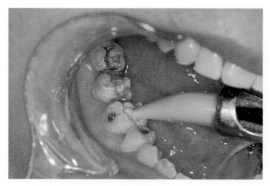

Fig. 5-150. Base cement inserted using a syringe. This is essentially a Class 1 cavity so a matrix is not used.

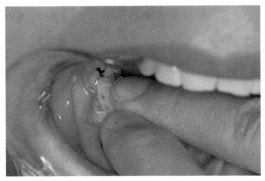

Fig. 5-151. A matrix strip is inserted and adequate finger pressure applied. This is necessary to assure adhesion of the cement.

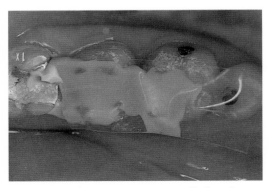

Fig. 5-152. After pressure was applied and setting completed.

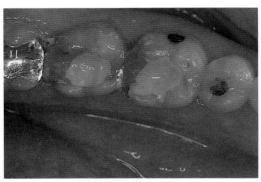

Fig. 5-153. The excess cement is removed, and by accurately exposing the cavity margins, establishing the margins when the cavity is prepared a second time will be easy. The patient is sent home like this.

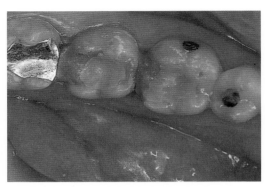

Fig. 5-154. How the patient returned to the clinic. Three weeks had passed, but the condition of the cement is hardly changed from before.

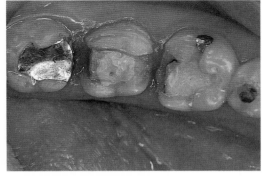

Fig. 5-155. Cavity preparation completed. The first molar is a MO with the mesiobuccal cusp coverage. The second molar is a MOD with complete buccal cusp coverage. It is of course also possible to restore this with full-coverage cast crowns.

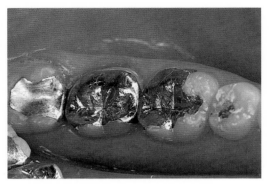

Fig. 5-156. Luting the cast restorations. The second molar looks like a full-coverage crown from the occlusal, but it only has cusp coverage.

Section 6: Glass Ionomer Cement Containing Metal Cements With Silver: Its Use For Bases

Koichi Narikawa, Benji Fujii
Department of Restorative Dentistry
Osaka Dental College

Today, we may have reached the point at which cement designed for use as a base can be clinically evaluated in its own right. Still, it is difficult for glass ionomer cement to rise above the properties of its basic components. To improve that aspect of the cement, the idea of sintering glass ionomers with silver and then having amalgam alloy added to the glass ionomer cement was born. The addition of amalgam alloy to cement itself was envisioned as early as zinc phosphate cement was used for bases since its resistance to cutting then becomes greater than the cement itself, and its strength was also presumed to be superior.

But according to reports from a meeting on restoratives, almost no improvement in strength is seen when silver is sintered with glass ionomer or when amalgam alloy is added. The same result was seen with regard to the adhesion to dentin. Therefore, there are not any particular advantages to this formulation other than radiopacity, even in clinical experiments.

Cement with sintered silver is marketed by ESPE Co. of Germany. The product shines like amalgam when polished after placement. However, it is found clinically that the margins fracture easily, and there is a concern that the marginal seal may be inferior.

The technique of mixing amalgam alloy into glass ionomer cement in the clinic has been made public, but we are still investigating the basic properties of this material in our department, and many points are still unclear. This cement becomes black when mixed, and the shine of the sintered cement is not seen even when it is polished. According to our experiments, various interesting phenomenon can be seen depending on the amount of alloy added, but it will be awhile before we can present a summary of the results.

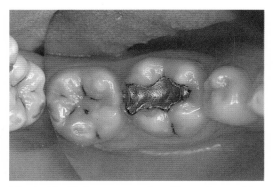

Fig. 5-157. Before restoration. Extensive caries beneath amalgam including the distal of mandibular left first molar. Shallow caries also on mesial and distal of left second molar.

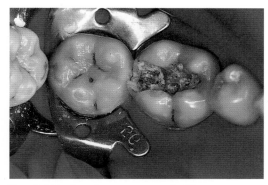

Fig. 5-158. Amalgam removed. There was a strong feeling that rather than being recurrent caries from the margin, they were caries left when it was previously restored.

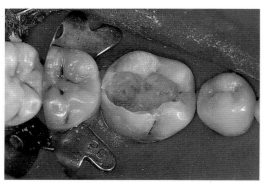

Fig. 5-159. Caries removed. Distal enamel fractured. At this point the design of the cavity is established, and if it is recorded in the chart, there is no confusion when the cavity is prepared.

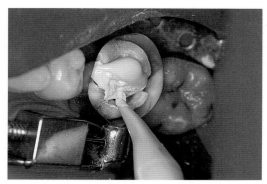

Fig. 5-160. An amalgam-type of matrix band is used on the first molar, *Chelon-Silver* in inserted with a syringe, and pressure is applied.

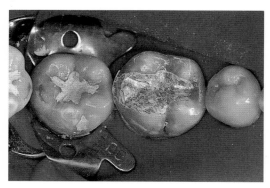

Fig. 5-161. An amalgam base (foundation) is placed in the second molar, and the finishing of the *Chelon-Silver* on the first molar is completed. The shine of the first molar is similar to that of the amalgam restorations.

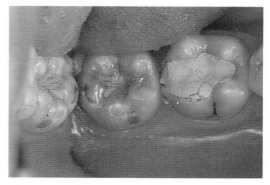

Fig. 5-162. Patient returned to the clinic 2 months later. The cement base on the first molar was subjected to heavy occlusal stresses and fractured. Some of the shine is also gone. There is also the danger that the bulk of the material fractured.

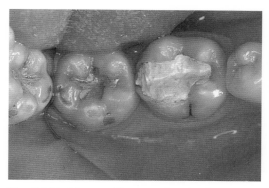

Fig. 5-163. Along with removing the fractured section that day, the cement base was refinished. The shine still did not come back.

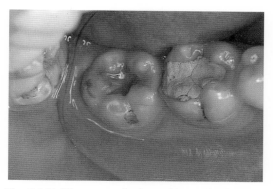

Fig. 5-164. Three months later (5 months from base being placed), same area fractured, and a new cavity preparation required.

CASE 2

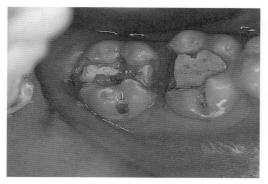

Fig. 5-165. Cavity preparation completed. The first molar is a DO with distobuccal cusp coverage. The pulpal wall and the axial walls are almost all in cement base. The second molar is a MOD. The base is polyacrylate cement.

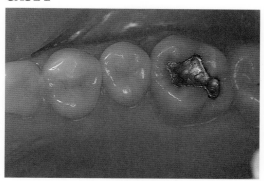

Fig. 5-166. Maxillary right first molar, second premolar and first premolar before restoration. Interpoximal caries were confirmed on the bitewing radiographs.

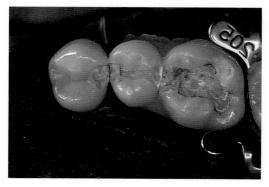

Fig. 5-167. Removal of the amalgam restoration and detection of interproximal caries.

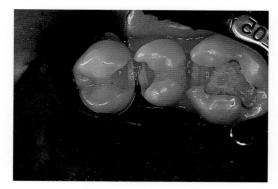

Fig. 5-168. Caries removal completed. Extensive, deep caries existed on all of the interproximal surfaces. If possible, placement of the rubber dam starting with caries removal is desirable.

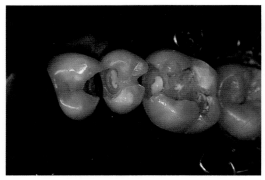

Fig. 5-169. Subbase of calcium hydroxide (dycal) placed in the deepest areas (indirect pulp cap). A subbase was also placed in the distal of the first premolar.

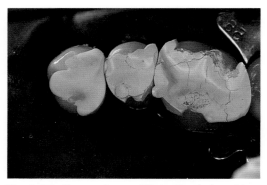

Fig. 5-170. Cement base of *Ketac-Bond* placed in the first premolar, and base of *Chelon-Silver* placed in the premolars. After insertion and application of pressure.

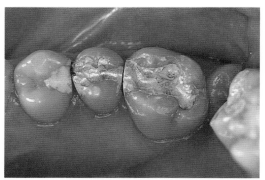

Fig. 5-171. Excess cement is removed with a round bur, and cavity margins are clearly exposed. A shine like that of amalgam can be seen after finishing the *Chelon-Silver*.

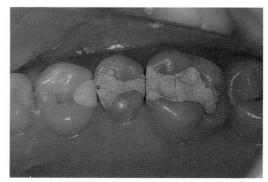

Fig. 5-172. Patient returned to the clinic one month later. The shine on the *Chelon-Silver* has disappeared, and a tendency for the center of the occlusal surface of the first molar to fracture can be seen.

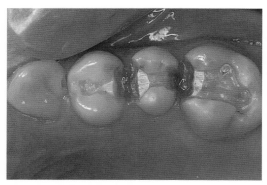

Fig. 5-173. Cavity preparation completed. All of the axial surfaces are formed in the cement base.

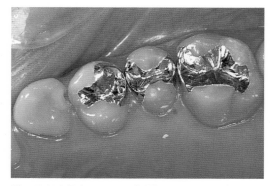

Fig. 5-174. Inlays seated. The patient does not complain of strange sensations such as pain with cold water.

CHAPTER VI

LONG-TERM
OBSERVATIONS

LONG TERM OBSERVATIONS ON GLASS IONOMER CEMENT

Sueo Saito
Department of Restorative Dentistry
Tokyo Medical and Dental College

Case Significance

Clinicians who were afraid of pulpal injury from resin-based restorative materials used glass ionomer cement as a tooth-colored restorative material safe for the pulp. They had high initial expectations, but the cement's applicability as a restorative material was mired in postoperative problems such as the appearance of white spots, dislodgement, and fracture. Still, the majority of these poor outcomes were caused by poor management of the material clinically, and the desirable properties could have been obtained had the proper chemical reaction (setting reaction) occurred. It became clear that these less-than-optimal properties resulted from moisture, such as saliva, entering into the setting reaction, especially in the initial period.

The cases presented here show results over a 10-year period. In general, observation of clinical cases, even now, is essentially a comparison of the successful and unsuccessful cases. I should also mention that I don't believe that the results of trial restorative materials are very meaningful. The reason for this is that the success or failure of the restoration by a trial material is largely due to: (1) selection of appropriate cases, (2) placement techniques, (3) powder-to-liquid ratio and mixing conditions, preparation of materials, and factors relating to the manufacturing of the product. The easier it is to reproduce the material's ideal (extraoral) properties in the mouth, the less effect technique will have on the outcome, and conversely, the more that various conditions in the mouth affect the setting reaction, the more strongly technique controls the outcome after treatment. The first on the list of topics to be discussed is that glass ionomer cement is a material affected by technique.

Then what can we learn from purported "clinical results"? The causative factors behind varying clinical results are what we must search out. If there are symptoms of discomfort, the causes should be sought out, and if results are good, the reasons for success must be probed. From such a process, we should be able to glean which cases are appropriate, then develop techniques for various types of cavities. That is, the observation of clinical results provides data for achieving better results, and not for a final evaluation of the material itself.

To achieve this purpose, every step must be conscious — from preparation of the material to placement technique, and so on. This means that research spread among numerous clinicians has certain limitations. For the results presented here, I was normally the clinician.

From observing the clinical results that I obtained with glass ionomer cement, I would say that the appropriate cases for glass ionomer cement were mostly those in which there was a fear that adverse pulpal reaction would occur with composite resin. Another condition was that the restoration be in a region which did not bear heavy external forces. In contrast to this, inappropriate cases were those in which composite resin could be used without fear of pulpal reaction. Even on the occlusal surface of molars, if glass ionomer is used within limits and good results are obtained, then it is perfectly fine to use. I would be delighted if you would carefully examine these as cases which obtained either positive or negative results, even though they do not have a lot of relevance on paper.

Case 1: Clinical Investigation of Abrasion Resistance and Adhesion

In order to investigate the extent of adhesion to enamel and the effect of toothbrush abrasion on the surface, *Fuji Ionomer Type II* was applied to the labial of the maxillary left canine, without any pretreatment, only with drying. A groove was cut, and the limits of the adhesion and the extent of the abrasion were investigated. The experiment was started in June 1977. The subject brushed with strong horizontal strokes, and this canine provided rigorous testing conditions for a toothbrush abrasion test (Fig. 6-1). As intraoral photographs would not show distinct details of the groove, the abrasion was compared by using the surface of stone models as shown in Figures 6-2, 6-3, and 6-4. The depth of the groove was 0.2-0.3 mm, and there was a lot less abrasion than imagined at the start of the experiment. The cement of course has not been lost, and the experiment still continues today.

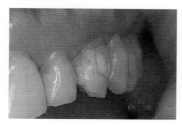

Fig. 6-1. Intraoral observation of experiment; (old *Fuji Type II*) applied to buccal surface of maxillary left first molar to test bond strength and abrasion resistance.

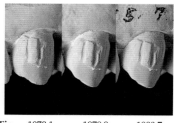
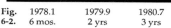

| Fig. | 1978.1 | 1979.9 | 1980.7 |
| 6-2. | 6 mos. | 2 yrs | 3 yrs |

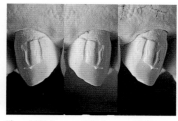

| Fig. | 1981.3 | 1982.5 | 1984.3 |
| 6-3. | 4 yrs | 5 yrs | 6 yrs |

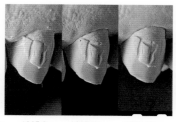

| Fig. | 1985.9 | 1987.10 | 1988.10 |
| 6-4. | 8 yrs | 10 yrs | 11 yrs |

Figs. 6-2, 6-3, 6-4. Stone models from 6 months to 11 years. Corners of groove edges started to wear at about 4 years and became rounded, and the roundness increased with time. At 10 years a section from central cervical region fractured and was lost. But the groove on the surface did not disappear even with 11+ years of heavy abrasion.

Case 2: Outcome 10 Years After Restoration of a Cervical Abrasion Lesion (Restored at the same time with macrofilled resin)

The cervical region of the maxillary right canine was restored with *Fuji Ionomer Type II* in May 1978. On the same day, a lining was placed in the maxillary right first premolar, and it was restored with macrofilled resin. Ten years later, the surface of the composite resin is discolored (stained), and it can be inferred from the condition of the gingiva that brushing has not been very hard. Light abrasion was found in the outward appearance of the glass ionomer cement on the maxillary first molar, but it was so limited that it was hardly detectable in the photo, and no stain line was seen around the margin of the restoration. Clinically, no need was found to replace the restoration. Furthermore, craze lines did not appear even with strong drying.

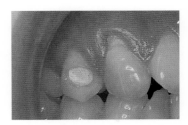

Fig. 6-5. Cavity preparation completed. Base placed for composite resin restoration in maxillary right first premolar.

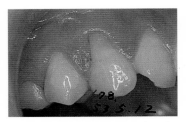

Fig. 6-6. Finishing completed 1 week after filling.

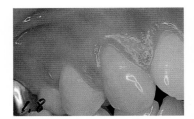

Fig. 6-7. 1 year, 8 months after restoration.

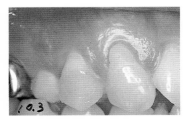

Fig. 6-8. Maxillary right canine, *Fuji Ionomer Type II*. Maxillary right first premolar 10 years, 3 months after restoring with macrofilled composite resin.

Case 3: Results After 9 Yrs. and 9 Mos. for *Fuji Ionomer Type II* in Saucer-Shaped Lesions in Mandibular Anterior Teeth

(Results of light water sensitivity)

Fuji Ionomer Type II was placed in shallow saucer-shaped cavities in the cervical lesions on the mandibular anterior teeth in November 1987. This also served as an adhesive experiment. This case shows, though periodic observation, that the left canine and lateral did not have any water sensitivity, but in the photo it was found that the left central had light water sensitivity under the drying test. However, this extent of water sensitivity (a chalky white spot did not occur) did not have a large effect clinically over time in this position. Additionally, at three years, no craze lines appeared even when the restoration was dried thoroughly.

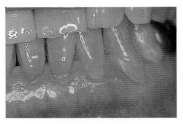

Fig. 6-9. Mandibular anterior teeth before cavity preparation. *Fuji Ionomer Type II* restoration will be placed with the teeth almost in this condition.

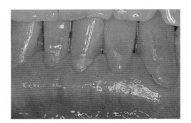

Fig. 6-10. November 1987, 1 week after restoration completed, dried. White spots of light water sensitivity can be seen on the central incisors, but no white spots are seen on left canine and lateral incisor.

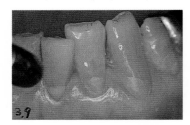

Fig. 6-11. At 3 years and 9 months. No craze lines appear even with strong drying.

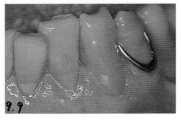

Fig. 6-12. At 9 years and 9 months. An extremely favorable result is shown, with almost no abrasion seen.

Fig. 6-13. Varnish isolation. A case from before the finishing period was established. Com-

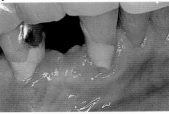

Case 4: Results of a Water-Sensitive Restoration and of a Replaced Restoration Over 8 Years

A clinical case from 1976, the very early period before isolation by varnish was established, when cases with water sensitivity were replaced. This was before powder-to-liquid ratio and clinical shade guides were established. Still, time has passed without any effect on the pulp.

Air bubbles from the interior were exposed by abrasion, the extent of which can be estimated from changes in bubbles shape. Neither the material nor the techniques were mature then, but finding neither stain lines nor fractures makes this case a reference.

pletely water-sensitive and one section has fractured and been lost. At that time I, too, thought that clinical use material was impossible.

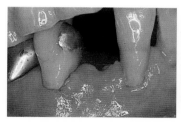

Fig 6-14. Immediately after redoing the restoration because varnish isolation technique had been established.

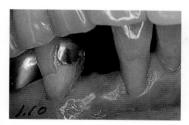

Fig. 6-15. At 1 year and 10 months, air bubbles from the interior appear on the surface because of the abrasion.

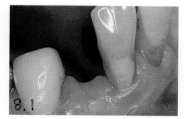

Fig. 6-16. At 8 years and 1 month. The extent of the abrasion can be estimated by changes in the edges and shape of the restoration since 1 year 10 months.

Case 5: Results 9 Years After Restoration of Proximal Root Caries

In this case, a tooth was restored with *Fuji Ionomer Type I* (luting) in 1976 before *Fuji Ionomer Type II* was produced. At that time, isolation with varnish had also not been perfected, and cocoa butter was used for isolation. Because glass ionomer cement is a restorative material which could be retained in the root region, and also since pulpal injury by composite resin was feared, this case was restored with glass ionomer cement. At present, even 10 years later, no treatment of any kind has been needed.

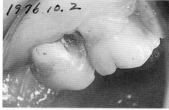

Fig. 6-17. Caries extending from the mesial of the maxillary right second molar onto the root.

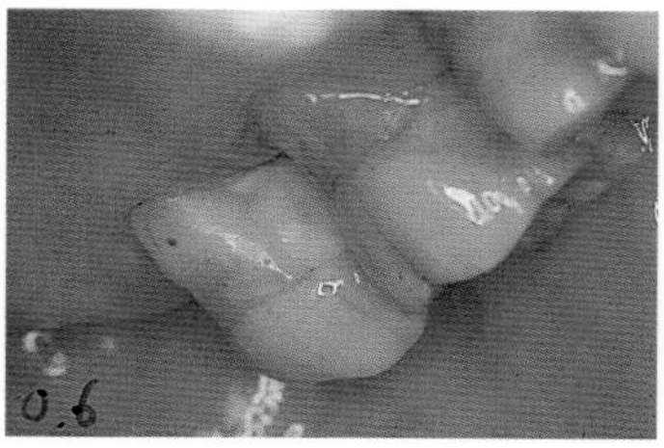

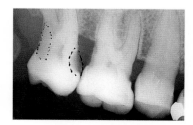

Fig. 6-18. *Fuji Ionomer Type II* restoration at 6 months.

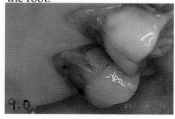

Fig. 6-19. The mesial and distal of the second molar have been restored, but because they are not radiopaque they appear translucent. This is an appropriate case for glass ionomer cement.

Fig. 6-20. 9 years after. Surface roughness is conspicuous, and may arise from weakened properties due to water sensitivity. However, the objective was accomplished.

Note: It was demonstrated later that trying to isolate with cocoa butter was not useful at all. Therefore, this case can be regarded as having had a lot of water sensitivity. Nevertheless, an obvious defect did not occur since it is in an area with no external forces.

Note: Modern *Fuji Ionomer Type II* is radiopaque.

Case 6: Case 11 Years After Treatment. Properties Lowered Due to Decreased Powder in Powder-to-Liquid Ratio.
(Compare abrasion with results of using *Palakav*.)

This is a restorative case of *Fuji Ionomer Type II* in June 1977, in the very early period of glass ionomer, and in order to adjust the color, the cement was mixed with less powder (liquid 1 : powder 1.8) than the standard liquid to powder ratio of 1:2.2. (Increasing the liquid increased the transparency and the color

improved.) At six years, abrasion was seen in the labial surface of the canine, and at 11 years, it became necessary to replace the restoration. However, in hte interproximal region, there was no abrasion, and stain lines were also not visible. In this case the 12 year outcome of using *Palakav* can also be seen at the same time.

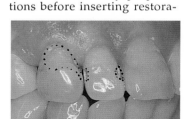

Fig. 6-21. Dotted lines on maxillary right canine and lateral incisor show cavity preparations before inserting restorative material. White restored areas on labial of right lateral and central incisors restored with *Palakav* (at about 1 year).

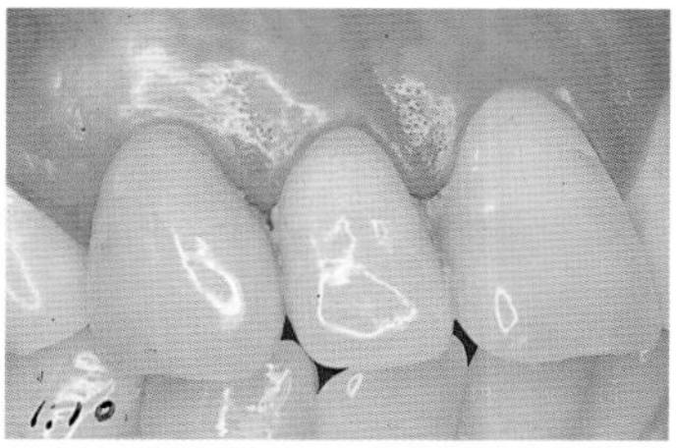

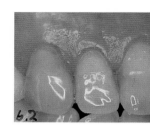

Fig. 6-22. 1 year and 10 months after restoring with *Fuji Ionomer Type II*. Clean, attractive restorations. (Debris and plaque between canine, lateral and central cover up the cleanness.)

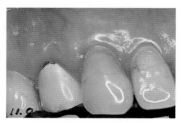

Fig. 6-23. At 6 years and 2 months. Abrasion on the cervical region of the canine is seen but there is no particular change in the interproximal region. Abrasion of the section restored with *Palakav* can also be seen at the same time.

Fig. 6-24. At 11 years. Canine restored again because of increased abrasion with gingival recession. Abrasion of *Palakav* clear. A stain line can be seen on the interproximal near the contact point. No other discoloration or abrasion, and almost no need for restoring them again.

Note: *Palakav* is a composite resin which has a MMA spheroid filler and bonds to dentin.

Note: Properties of *Palakav*: Compressive strength:700-1200kg/cm², resistance to toothbrush abrasion 0.01 mm.

Cases 7, 8, 9. Applicability for Lingual Pits in Anterior Teeth, Occlusal Surfaces of Primary Teeth, and Hypersensitive Root Surfaces

The use of glass ionomer cement as a permanent restoration on the occlusal surface of permanent teeth cannot be considered because of its basic properties, but cavities in permanent teeth which are limited to the pits on the buccal and lingual which do not receive many occlusal forces, and root caries as well as the occlusal surfaces of primary teeth where even masticatory forces are weak, are good

cases for application of glass ionomer cement because there is no fear of pulpal stimulation or secondary caries. Furthermore, the restorative procedures are not complicated. In these cases, there is little demand for esthetics, so by mixing in a little extra powder, an improvement in the properties and a shortening of water-sensitivity time were able to be achieved.

CASE 7

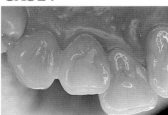

Fig. 6-25. 5 years after restoring a carious lingual pit extremely close to the dental pulp. No recurrent caries and good prognosis.

CASE 9

Treatment result of a case of hypersensitivity on exposed root surface.

CASE 8

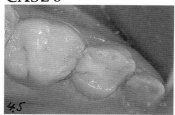

Fig. 6-26. Class 2 cavities in primary molars 4 years and 5 months after restoration. A step can be seen from abrasion of margins, but no secondary caries detected.

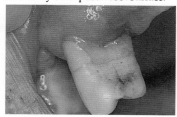

Fig. 6-27. Hypersensitive root surface as commonly seen in the elderly. Surface layer removed, *Fuji Ionomer Type II* applied, and hypersensitivity disappeared.

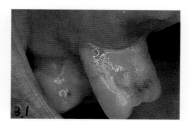

Fig. 6-28. At 3 years and 1 month. Hygiene is not good (plaque on surface), but hypersensitivity has not returned.

Case 10: Case Where Restoration With Composite Resin Was Difficult

The cavity preparation of caries on the buccal surface of maxillary molars and the filling procedures are extremely difficult in this area. It is impossible to completely carry out all of the adhesive procedures such as isolation and, for certain, etching (indispensable to prevent symptoms of discomfort after treatment with a composite resin restoration). Also, lining cannot be placed adequately when it is required. If glass ionomer cement is used, it is possible to restore without the need to use a liner and with no fear regarding the dental pulpal tissues.

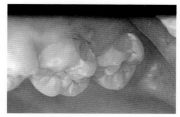

Fig. 6-29. 15-year-old girl. Caries on labial of maxillary left first and second molars. Cavity preparation completed.

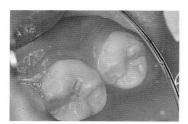

Fig. 6-30. Restoration of first and second molars completed with *Fuji Ionomer Type II.* 1 month after, there was no pulpal reaction.

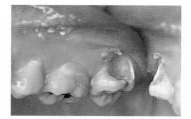

Fig. 6-31. 17-year-old boy. Exposed cavity on labial of maxillary left second molar. *Fuji Ionomer Type II* filled directly over direct pulp cap.

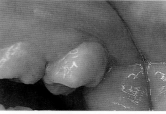

Fig. 6-32. No pain after treatment, good prognosis.

The Ideal Restorative Material and Glass Ionomer Cement

From the results of clinical and intraoral experiments over 30 years ago, a theory that the basic condition of restorative materials should be that they "adapt well to the tooth" was reached. What properties, precisely, does this "adapt well to tooth" indicate?

I. Essential biologic aspects:
  1) Biocompatibility with tooth
II. As physical properties:
  1) Hydrophilic
  2) Adhesion to tooth structure
  3) Wets tooth structure well
  4) Physical strength similar to that of tooth
  5) Dimension change is small when setting
  6) Thermal expansion is similar to tooth structure

So let's take a look at how today's restorative materials today fulfill these properties.

1. Gold inlays have sufficient physical strength and thermal expansion but are not hydrophilic or adhesive, nor do they have good wetting properties. Nonetheless, gold inlays have a good clinical outcome because luting cement which adapts to tooth is introduced between the tooth and the restoration.

2. For composite resins, biocompatibility and the hydrophilic properties are a shortcoming, and the dimensional changes on setting and wettability of tooth are bad when they are light-cured. The thermal expansion has been improved by adding filler, but it is still not good enough. However, composite resins show good clinical results because of the strong strength of adhesion. For this reason, great damage occurs when adequate adhesion cannot be obtained (Figs. 6-33, 6-34).

3. The physical strength of glass ionomer cement is a weak point and there are large individual differences also in the material's adhesion to dentin, but the adhesion to enamel is favorable. More than anything else, the strong points are the biocompatibility to tooth, hydrophilic properties, good wetting properties, and thermal expansion similar to that of tooth structure. From clinical results, it is felt that this is the restorative material which is the most "adapting to tooth" as stated earlier. However, due to the very important physical strength being inferior, at present it is necessary to avoid placing this material in an environment which is affected by strong external forces such as occlusal forces. If increases in properties in the future can be devised, this material releases fluoride and can be used for various new objectives, and good results can be expected.

(Sueo Saito)

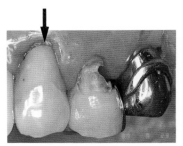

Fig. 6-33. Composite resin which does not bond to dentin in the cervical region of the maxillary left canine.

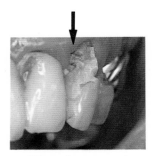

Fig. 6-34. When the composite resin was removed, it was clear that the caries underneath had spread out. This type of thing does not occur with glass ionomer cement.

CHAPTER VII

THE GLASS IN GLASS IONOMER CEMENT POWDERS

THE GLASS IN GLASS IONOMER CEMENT POWDERS

CHEMICAL COMPOSITION AND STRUCTURE

Nobuhiko Ogata
Toru Maeda
Takajiro Shimohira
Shigeru Katsuyama

If the history of the rapid progression in dental cements is reviewed, it can be seen that the chemical composition of glass ionomer cement powder was derived from silicate cement powder, which was created in 1902. The chemical composition in the early period of glass ionomer cements was an Na_2O - CaO - Al_2O_3 - SiO_2 type glass. Later, after CaO was changed to CaF_2, the use of Na_2O was discontinued and small quantities of P_2O_5 and NaF were added. The properties of the material were thereby markedly improved.[B32]

The composition of the original silicate cement powder is not much different from the powder used in today's glass ionomer cements and the properties of the powder itself have not changed much. However, glass ionomer cement powder has slightly less SiO_2, and is alkaline.

Basically, the core of the cement is formed from calcium fluoroaluminosilicate glasses. The relative content of silica, alumina, and fluoride cannot be viewed as a constant, as it varies according to manufacturer. There are also products which, depending on their intended use, have pigments or radiopaque agents added, or radiopaque components may be contained within the glass of the powder itself. Tannin fluoride agents may also be added. Furthermore, some products also contain components of the liquid, e.g., polyacrylic acid, in the powder as a polymer, but here we refer only to the composition of the glass itself.

The raw materials of the glass are basically silica (SiO_2), alumina (Al_2O_3), fluorite (CaF_2), sodium fluoride (NaF), and aluminum phosphate ($AlPO_4$). These raw materials are mixed in prescribed ratios, placed in a crucible, and melted at between 1000° and 1350°C. After the mixture has completely melted, the crucible is removed from the furnace, and the material is poured onto a room-temperature steel plate while still fluid. With sudden cooling in this manner, some distortion occurs, and it becomes easier to make a fine powder out of the material. Since the glass contains a relatively large amount of fluoride, the time it is held at a high temperature is kept as short as possible to reduce the loss of the volatile fluorides.

A relatively large particle size is acceptable for restorative or base cements, but particles as small as possible are desired for adhesives. Since the setting of the cement starts with the dissolution of the glass in polyacrylic acid, the speed of the setting reaction is thought to be proportional to the size of the glass powder. When the hardened material is observed with an electron microscope, many of the glass particles are left, and these glass pieces become a core dispersed within the matrix. Although at this point we cannot state quantitatively the extent to which the glass dissolves during setting, there is a range in the distribution of the particle sizes, and furthermore, the finer the particle the more it should be seen to dissolve. It has been reported that the core/matrix area ratio with an adhesive glass ionomer shown in scanning electron micrographs is 2:8 according to the image analyzer.[B33] It has also been reported that the quantity of remaining core for silicate cements using calcium fluoroaluminosilicate

Table 7-1. Chemical composition of sample glasses. (mole %)

	SiO_2	P_2O_5	Al_2O_3	CaF_2	NaF	LaF_3	CeF_3	ZrO_2	SrO	BaO	B_2O_3
G-200A	35.98	3.07	19.61	35.91	5.33						
G-200B	38.70	3.27	21.44	35.23	1.35						
G-237	49.51	4.18	20.85	25.46							
K-1	45.69		17.12	17.58	19.61						
K-2	45.62		21.18	9.70	23.50						
N-1	35.10	7.60	18.86	32.41	6.03						
N-3	43.47		18.30	38.23							
N-4	39.19		16.69	38.77	5.35						
N-6	40.00		23.77	30.78	5.45						
N-9	31.76	3.00	16.08	28.19	20.97						
N-10	27.17	3.04	16.26	32.32	21.21						
N-11	41.45	3.52	21.42	23.10	6.13	4.38					
N-12	31.80	3.60	30.62	23.40	6.20	4.40					
N-14	31.80	3.60	30.62	23.40	6.20		4.40				
N-15	32.10	3.60	30.90	23.60	6.20			3.60			
N-16	41.00		24.36	21.53	5.59				7.52		
N-17	40.40	2.02	20.90	31.00	5.50						
N-18	41.37	2.26	21.42	21.72	5.64				7.59		
N-19	42.02		24.97	22.07	5.73					5.21	
N-20	40.97		18.96	21.53	5.57					5.07	7.90
N-21	41.31	2.26	15.99	21.77	5.63					5.12	7.92
N-22	46.04	0.63	29.49	18.23	5.61						
N-23	44.42	0.64	27.22	22.11	5.61						
N-24	41.44		27.70	13.67	4.23	4.54			8.43		

glass is 80%.[B34] According to our research, the remaining core is about 25% to 52%, with a large range of values.[B35] This may have been due to inadequate mixing.

Examples of representative glass compositions are shown in Table 7-1, and the melting temperature, melting state, and type of precipitate are shown in Table 7-2. Ca, Al and F are very plentiful relative to normal glass. Because of this, the glasses take on an opal, semi-transparent or white, opaque appearance. This composition was chosen because one portion dissolves in polyacrylic acid, and the Ca^{2+} and Al^{3+} ions separate. These ions react with polyacrylic acid to form the hard matrix structure which is necessary to produce an acceptable cement.

Ions in the glass are divided into network-former cations, network-modifying cations, and network-former anions; Si^{4+} and Al^{3+} are suitable as network-former cations, while Ca^{2+}, Na^+ and other alkali or alkali earth ions are suitable network-modifying cations, and O^{2-} and F^- are suitable anions.

Silica glass is the simplest of all silicate glasses, with a structure in which the essential elements of the $(SiO_4)_n$ tetrahedra are linked three dimensionally, with all the Si^{4+} ions surrounded by four O^{2-} ions, and all O^{2-} ions attached to two Si^{4+} ions. A portion of the Si^{4+} in these positions is replaced with Al^{3+} and becomes aluminosilicate glass; this portion of the basic structure of the tetrahedron therefore becomes (AlO_4). To satisfy the requirement of electrical neutrality, P_2O_5 is sometimes added, and the substitution of $2Si^{4+} \longleftrightarrow Al^{3+} \bullet P^{5+}$ occurs. The more Al^{3+} is substituted for the Si^{4+}, the more the net-

Table 7-2. Melting state and precipitation crystals of experimental glasses.

	Fusion temp. (°C)	Melting state		Visual appearance after solidification	Precipitation crystals identified by x-ray diffraction (Cu K$_\alpha$)
		Viscosity	Fluidity		
G200A	1250	little	good	clear glass	CaF$_2$
G200B	1350	little	good	opal glass	CaF$_2$
G237	1350	some	good	clear glass	non-crystalline
K1	1000	some	good	white opaque	CaF$_2$
K2	950	little	good	white opaque	CaF$_2$
N1	1050	some	good	white opaque	non-crystalline
N3	1250	some	good	white opaque	CaF$_2$
N4	1250	little	good	white opaque	CaF$_2$
N6	1250	much	poor	white opaque	CaF$_2$
N9	900	some	good	white opaque	CaF$_2$
N10	900	some	good	white opaque	CaF$_2$
N11	1100	little	good	white opaque	CaF$_2$- LaF$_3$solid solution
N12	1300	little	poor	white opaque	α- Al$_2$O$_3$,CaF$_2$- LaF$_3$solid solution,(?)
N14	1300	much	poor	buff opaque	α- Al$_2$O$_3$,CaF$_2$- CeF$_3$solid solution
N15	1350	little	good	white opaque	α- Al$_2$O$_3$,CaF$_2$,(?)
N16	1300	little	good	white opaque	CaF$_2$
N17	1200	little	good	white opaque	CaF$_2$
N18	1250	little	good	white opaque	CaF$_2$
N19	1250	little	good	white opaque	CaF$_2$
N20	1250	little	good	white opaque	CaF$_2$
N21	1200	little	good	white opaque	CaF$_2$
N22	1300	much	poor	white opaque	α- Al$_2$O$_3$
N23	1250	little	poor	white opaque	α- Al$_2$O$_3$,CaF$_2$
N24	1300	little	poor	white opaque	CaF$_2$- LaF$_3$solid solution

Note: (?) Single phase not yet identified

work structure becomes unstable and resistance to chemicals is weakened, i.e., reactivity toward acid is increased. In this way, reactivity increases when Al$_2$O$_3$ is increased much, the melting temperature is markedly elevated and melting becomes difficult.

CaF$_2$, a flux, has been added to address these circumstances, and a structure which can easily be melted at economical temperatures below 1350°C has been made. The fusion temperature can be lowered not only with fluorides, but also with alkalis represented by Na and components for network formers like B$_2$O$_3$ and P$_2$O$_5$. However, components other than P$_2$O$_5$ are almost never used as glass components in this cement, probably because these components do not effectively elevate the strength of the cement. The selection of flux is extremely important since research results show that the strength of hardened cement using glass with much Na is markedly low.[B36]

The presence of excess CaF$_2$ induces either two-phase separation or crystal precipitation within the glass, and the glass becomes semi-transparent or opaque. The condition of crystal precipitation depends on the speed of cooling after melting. That is, if the substance is cooled quickly enough, there are few precipitation crystals, but if it is cooled slowly, an adequate quantity of crystals are

Table 7-3. Melting point and composition of SiO_2- Al_2O_3- CaF_2 three-component system glass.

Sample number	Chemical composition (mole %)			Fusion temp. (°C)	State of melting		Appearance
	SiO_2	Al_2O_3	CaF_2		Viscosity	Fluidity	
SAC 1	48.45	14.28	37.27	1350	little	good	white opaque
SAC 2	38.24	22.53	39.23	1350	little	good	separated into two phases
SAC 3	58.91	13.89	27.20	1300	some	pull-type	white opaque
SAC 4	49.53	21.89	28.58	1300	some	pull-type	white opaque
SAC 5	39.14	30.75	30.11	1300	much	poor	buff opaque
SAC 6	60.19	21.20	18.52	1350	much	poor	clear glass
SAC 7	50.66	29.85	19.49	1350	much	poor	white opaque

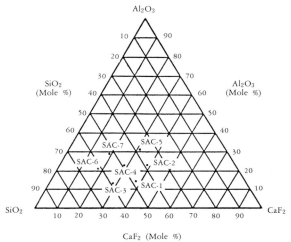

Fig. 7-1. SiO_2-Al_2O_3-CaF_2 system. Chemical composition of experimental glass.

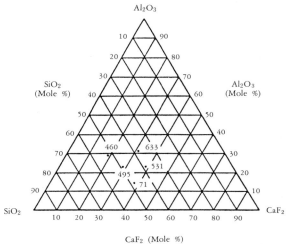

Fig. 7-2. Compressive strength of set cement using the SiO_2-Al_2O_3-CaF_2 system glass (Kgf/cm^2).

precipitated. For that reason, when cooled quickly on a steel plate, the surface of the molten mass as well as the portion contacting the steel plate will probably have few precipitation crystals. However, a large quantity of crystals will precipitate in the center of the molten mass, since it cools rather slowly. Making powder from this kind of molten mass should pose no problems, even if there are some glass particles with many precipitation crystals and some glass particles with few. This was confirmed with SEM observations of the hardened cement we made.[B37]

A SiO_2 - Al_2O_3 - CaF_2 Three-Component Glass System

We made an experimental glass with hardly any network modifying ions except Ca, and prepared a hardened cement mass. Table 7-3 shows the chemical composition, fusion temperature, and melting state of the glasses.

The mass was crushed with an agate mortar, and passed through a 325 mesh (44μ) sieve, making a powder. *Fuji Ionomer Type I* (GC Corp.) liquid was used with a powder-to-liquid ratio of 1.8. This was mixed, and a hardened cylinder of cement with a diameter of 6 mm was made, following the universal standard. After the samples were stored in 37°C distilled water for 24 hours, they were compressed with a cross-head speed of 1 mm/min, and compressive strength was determined.

The position of the chemical composition on a 3-component system diagram is shown for each material in Figure 7-1, and the distribution of the compressive strengths is shown in Figure 7-2. As shown in Figure 7-1, the range of the composition which hardened as cement is quite narrow, including only SAC 2, 4, 5, and 7. The other samples did not harden and were rich in SiO_2 and had little Al_2O_3. Also, hardened material which contained large amounts of both Al_2O_3 and SiO_2 dissolved away when it was stored in water. Judging from these results, it can be surmised that the optimal combina-

tion for the chemical composition of the glass would have as little SiO_2 as possible, and that the Al_2O_3 and CaF_2 would be in approximately equal proportions.

Since it is an alumino-silicate glass, the quantity of SiO_2 which forms the network structure is naturally limited, and is estimated to be approximately 30 mole percent. Therefore, glass with a chemical composition of greater than 30 mole percent SiO_2 was made, as shown in Table 7-1. The quantity of Al_2O_3 is as large as possible because previous research has shown that there is a tendency for strength to increase with higher Al_2O_3 content.

The G series on Table 7-1 is from Wilson et al's research, and the K series is cited from Kajiwara's research. Only the N series is of original compositions we created.

Melting State and Crystal Precipitation

The fusion temperature, melting state, visual appearance after setting, and type of crystal precipitation for the experimental glasses made by the method previously explained are shown in Table 7-2.

As can be imagined from the chemical composition, almost all of the CaF_2 that was contained in the glass precipitated as crystals. As a result, the glass was white and semi-transparent or opaque.

Also, x-ray diffraction showed that crystals of α- Al_2O_3 (corundum) precipitated for glasses containing large quantities of Al_2O_3. The visual appearance of the glasses and the results of x-ray diffraction did not always coincide. For example, there was a case when a CaF_2 peak was observed with x-ray diffraction even when visually clear glass was seen.

According to SEM observations, these fluoride crystals had all precipitated in the glass as minute droplets and were almost uniformly dispersed.

Figure 7-3 shows the distribution of the CaF_2 crystals which had precipitated in the glass, and Figure 7-4 shows their x-ray diffraction peaks. Visually, there were round

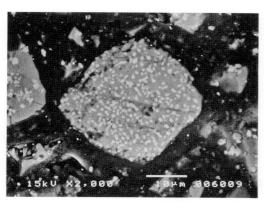

Fig. 7-3. CaF$_2$ crystals precipitated in the glass particles.

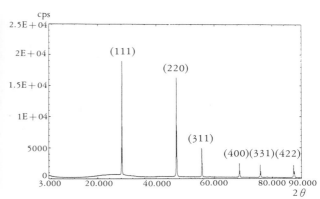

Fig. 7-4. X-ray diffraction peaks of CaF$_2$ precipitated in glass.

Table 7-4. Lattice constant of CaF$_2$ precipitated in the glass.

Peak No.	$2\theta°$	dÅ	I/I$_0$	(hkl)	a$_0$ (lattice constant) A
1	28.220	3.15968	100	(111)	5.47273
2	46.960	1.93330	86	(220)	5.46820
3	55.770	1.64886	27	(311)	5.46865
4	68.640	1.36620	14	(400)	5.46480
5	75.800	1.25395	13	(331)	5.46584
6	87.300	1.11594	12	(422)	5.46697
					Average 5.46786

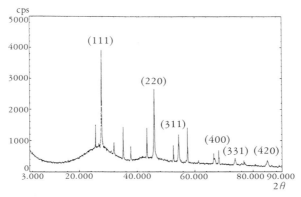

Fig. 7-5. X-ray diffraction peaks of sample N12.

droplets, but the x-ray diffraction peaks were sharp, and from this finding it can be concluded that these crystals are probably almost perfect. The size of the unit lattice is shown in Table 7-4. Since it is a value extremely close to the standard value of $a_0 = 5.46305$ Å, the crystals are probably almost pure CaF_2.

If rare earth metal fluorides are added and melted, the rare earth elements go into solid solution in CaF_2, and it seems as if the rare earth elements do not exist in the glass composition. In samples N11, 12, 14, and 24, the La^{3+} and Ce^{3+} ions always replaced the Ca^{2+} site in CaF_2. The peaks of x-ray diffraction for sample N12 are shown in Figure 7-5. If the size of the unit cell is determined from each of the diffraction peaks of CaF_2, $a_0 = 5.59299$ Å, as shown in Table 7-5, and is much greater than the standard value. The same tendency was seen when the CeF_3 in N14 was added.

La^{3+} and Ce^{3+} both have ionic radii slightly greater than Ca^{2+}, and the unit cell becomes larger for their substitution. This confirms the fact that precipitation crystals form a solid solution.

SEM observations were made to see how this kind of solid solution formation affects the visual appearance of the crystals (Fig. 7-6). The results confirmed that by becoming a solid solution, the dimension of the droplets of the crystals definitely became smaller. Since these were submicron particles of less than 1μm, the scattering power of the precipitate was restricted in the hardened cement, and as a result, the transparency should have increased. Therefore, the diameter of the dispersion is close to 1μm, because there is a maximum ability to scat-

Table 7-5. X-ray diffraction of sample N12.

Peak No.	$2\theta°$	d Å	I/I_0	CaF_2-LaF_3 solid solution (hkl)	a_0	α-Al_2O_3 (hkl)
1	25.540	3.48484	39			(012)
2	27.580	3.23153	100	(111)	5.59717	
3	31.040	2.87875	18			?
4	31.980	2.79625	25			?
5	35.100	2.55451	37			(104)
6	37.740	2.38166	21			?
7	43.320	2.08693	37			(113)
8	45.840	1.97789	68	(220)	5.59432	
9	52.520	1.74096	22			(024)
10	54.360	1.68630	31	(311)	5.59282	
11	57.460	1.60247	37			(116)
12	61.240	1.51231	10			?
13	66.480	1.40524	16			(124)
14	66.720	1.40077	12			?
15	68.180	1.37429	18	(400)(?)		(030)
16	73.820	1.28261	12	(311)	5.59077	
17	76.820	1.23982	10			(1010)
18	80.700	1.18971	7			?
19	84.920	1.14103	10	(420)	5.58988	
20	86.440	1.12482	6			?
21	88.960	1.09936	6			?
				Average a 5.59299Å		Average a_0 4.76068Å c_0 13.02583Å

Note:Single phase not yet identified

ter. Minutization of the droplets by the formation of this solid solution is probably also desirable for appropriate visual appearance of the cement with respect to tooth structure.

When the results in Tables 7-1 and 7-2 are compared, the crystal precipitation of α-Al_2O_3 (corundum) in glass containing more than 27 mole percent of Al_2O_3 is confirmed. For example, the x-ray diffraction peaks obtained from test sample N12 is shown in Fig. 7-5. A large portion of the peaks which do not conform to the Miller indices are appropriate for diffraction from α-Al_2O_3. The size of the unit cell of α-Al_2O_3 as determined by each peak is $a_o = 4.76068$ Å, and $c_o = 13.02583$ Å. Since the standard values are a_o - 4.758 Å, and $c_o = 12.991$ Å, these precipitated crystals are almost pure corundum crystals. Table 7-5 summarizes the x-ray diffraction results of sample N12. Some peaks from samples which could not be identified are included.

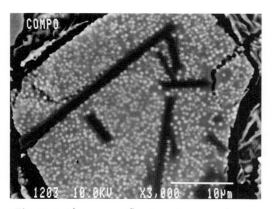

Fig. 7-6. Electron reflection image of sample N12.

When the precipitated α-Al_2O_3 was observed visually with SEM, all crystals were needle-shaped with a width of approximately 1μm and a length of several μm to 10 μm. The needle-shaped crystals are shown in Fig. 7-6. They are extremely large compared to those of CaF_2. Since the kind of needle-shaped crystal is distributed unevenly in the glass particles, a reinforcing effect can be expected. However, the reinforce-

ment of the hardened cement may not be directly affected.

An Empirical Formula

There are more ingredients forming glass than other substances, as seen in Table 7-1. The proportion of each ingredient is shown as both weight percent and as mole percent. When comparing the chemical composition of silicate glass with that of silicate minerals in order to make analogies, it is important to determine the empirical formula from the mole percent. For example, orthoclase, a mineral of the earth's crust, is $K_2O \cdot Al_2O_3 \cdot 6\ SiO_2$, but it is K_2O; 12.5, Al_2O_3; 12.5, SiO_2; 75, as mole percent. This becomes $K(AlSi_3)O_8$ when changed to an empirical formula, with the network-former cation groups indicated within the parentheses, the alkali placed on the left side as the network-modifier ions, and the anions placed on the right. The three-dimensional network of the linked $(AlSi_3)O_8$ tetrahedra is depicted in this formula, and it can seen that the K^+ ion is placed between the network structure. That is, K^+ compensates for the electrical charge deficiency from the Al^{3+} replacing the Si^{4+} position. If the glass structure is shown as an empirical formula of minerals in this way, analogies can be made even though to a certain extent the composition of the glass is complex.

Empirical formulas for representative glasses are shown in Table 7-6. Here, the network-former cation is indicated in the parentheses on the left, and the total of the coefficients was made to equal 1.00. The parentheses on the right indicate the fluorides of the precipitation crystals, and the modifying cations are indicated outside the parentheses. The figure in the lower right of each element indicates the relative number of each atom.

When P^{5+} is included in the network-former cations, electrical compensation of $P^{5+} + Al^{3+} \rightarrow 2Si^{4+}$ occurs within the network structure, and only Al^{3+} and Si^{4+} are considered network-former cations. The results of

Table 7-6. Empirical formulas of representative glasses.

Sample No.	(network former cation*) modifying cation and network former anion {precipitation crystal}
N6	$(Si_{0.457}Al_{0.543})$ $Na_{0.062}O_{1.782}F_{0.062}$ $\{CaF_2\}_{0.352}$
N9	$(Si_{0.454}P_{0.086}Al_{0.460})$ $Na_{0.300}O_{1.813}F_{0.300}$ $\{CaF_2\}_{0.403}$
N11	$(Si_{0.454}P_{0.077}Al_{0.469})$ $Na_{0.067}O_{1.804}F_{0.067}$ $\{(CaF_2)_{0.253} (LaF_3)_{0.048}\}$
N12	$(Si_{0.317}P_{0.072}Al_{0.611})$ $Na_{0.062}O_{1.731}F_{0.061}$ $\{(CaF_2)_{0.234} (LaF_3)_{0.044}\}$
N24	$(Si_{0.428}Al_{0.572})$ $Na_{0.044}Sr_{0.087}O_{1.801}F_{0.044}$ $\{(CaF_2)_{0.141} (LaF_3)_{0.047}\}$
G200A	$(Si_{0.443}P_{0.075}Al_{0.482})$ $Na_{0.066}O_{1.797}F_{0.066}$ $\{CaF_2\}_{0.441}$

*Total is 1.000

Table 7-7. Comparison of the network former cation of each sample glass.

Sample No.	Comparison of network former cations (Substituted $P^{5+}+Al^{3\pm} \to 2Si^{4+}$)
N6	$(Si_{0.46}-Al_{0.54}) \to (Si_{0.46} < Al_{0.54})$
N9	$(Si_{0.45} \ P_{0.09} \ Al_{0.46}) \to (Si_{0.67} > Al_{0.37})$
N11	$(Si_{0.45} \ P_{0.08} \ Al_{0.47}) \to (Si_{0.61} > Al_{0.39})$
N12	$(Si_{0.32} \ P_{0.07} \ Al_{0.61}) \to (Si_{0.46} < Al_{0.54})$
N24	$(Si_{0.43}- \ Al_{0.57}) \to (Si_{0.43} < Al_{0.57})$
G200A	$(Si_{0.44} \ P_{0.08} \ Al_{0.48}) \to (Si_{0.60} > Al_{0.40})$

this kind of substitution are shown in Table 7-7. N6, N12, and N24 have less Si and Al, and all of the others have more Si than Al. If there is less Si than Al, the Al-O-Al bridge becomes the network structure, and this makes an unstable structure. It is thought that when α-Al_2O_3 crystals precipitate, the total energy of the system becomes lower.

The results of Table 7-2 support the above-mentioned structure. That is, α-Al_2O_3 precipitate was found to comprise a large portion of the samples which contained less Si and Al. Therefore, even if Al_2O_3 content is increased to elevate the strength of the hardened cement, Al_2O_3 is not contained in the glass structure beyond some point, and we must recognize the fact that it precipitates as α-Al_2O_3. The limit is likely about Si $\fallingdotseq$ Al.

Strength and Composition

Generally it is said that the strength of set cement depends on the strength of the core itself, and it is desirable to use as strong a core as possible. Since the core of glass ionomer cement is unreacted, left-over glass, it is imagined that strong cement can be obtained by have the strength of the glass itself as high as possible. The details of the structure of the glasses are not as clear as that of the crystals. Therefore, even though the connection between the strength of the crystals and the structure is clearly explained in great detail, there is almost no theoretical explanation for the strength of the glass at present.

There are numerous chemical compositions for regular glass, and all components can be separated into network former, and network modifier, etc. according to the function of the structure of each component. It is thus possible to draw an image of the structure of glass to a certain extent by dividing the components in this way. However, it is extremely difficult to predict strength even if this kind of structural image is used.

Recent studies in this area have produced the following range of articles. Lowenstein has reported that the logarithm of field strength of cations contained in the glass is

Table 7-8. Relative weight, atomic packing density (V_t) and compressive strength of set glass ionomer cement for sample glasses.

	V_i/M	ρ (density, 21℃)	V_t {$=\rho(V_i/M)$}	compressive strength kg/cm² (24h)
G200A	0.2111	2.7760	0.5860	862
G-200B	0.2120	2.7905	0.5916	918
G-237	0.2166	2.6668	0.5776	347
K-1	0.2146	2.8860	0.5508	345
K-2	0.2162	2.5281	0.5466	626
N-1	0.2144	2.8860	0.6188	748
N-3	0.2102	2.7866	0.5857	540
N-4	0.2191	2.7369	0.5723	357
N-6	0.2109	2.7817	0.5867	900
N-9	0.2113	2.5930	0.5479	130
N-10	0.2096	2.6657	0.5587	74※
N-11	0.2045	2.8594	0.5847	442
N-12	0.2032	3.0215	0.6139	1013
N-14	0.2002	2.9972	0.6000	702
N-15	0.2038	2.9233	0.6090	780
N-16	0.2022	2.8470	0.5757	751
N-17	0.2124	2.7330	0.5805	713
N-18	0.2036	2.8430	0.5788	660
N-19	0.1891	2.8740	0.5436	735
N-20	0.2066	2.7301	0.5640	761
N-21	0.1965	2.7156	0.5336	631
N-22	0.2150	2.6161	0.5624	750
N-23	0.2139	2.7086	0.5794	664
N-24	0.1873	3.0518	0.5716	646
SAC-1	0.2131	2.7286	0.5815	71※
SAC-2	0.2091	2.7417	0.5733	531
SAC-3	0.2156	2.5900	0.5584	did not harden
SAC-4	0.2134	2.6729	0.5704	495
SAC-5	0.2110	2.8424	0.6084	633
SAC-6	0.2176	2.6160	0.5692	dissolved during storage in water
SAC-7	0.2153	2.6860	0.5783	460

※This was an exceptional hardened material, showing destruction with an extremely large amount of deformation when compressed.

proportional to the Young's modulus of glass; this was recognized experimentally in a large range of silicate glasses.[B38] Makishima et al have conducted an experiment of theoretically determining the Young's modulus from the dissociation energy of the bond between atoms forming the glass, and the Pauling ion radius.[B39,40] Anderson et al,[B41] Soga et al,[B42] and Bridge, et al[B43] have also done similar research. Theoretically derived equations for the calculation of Young's modulus of glasses is suggested from the models proposed by each of the researchers.

There is one common finding among all these models, and that is that the elastic moduli of glass is proportional to the atomic packing density as well as the atomic interaction force constants. At this point, it is dif-

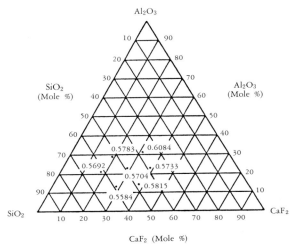

Fig. 7-7. SiO_2-Al_2O_3-CaF_2 system. Atomic packing density of sample glass.

ficult to estimate the constant of the work force between atoms, but it is possible to calculate the atomic packing density.

For example, Makishima's method is as follows. Suppose a glass is indicated by M_mO_n, and the Pauling's atomic radii of cations and anions as r_m and r_o. The packing factor V_i of the oxide components is determined from the following formula.

$V_i = (4\pi/3) \cdot N \cdot (m \cdot r_m^3 + n \cdot r_o^3)$ cc/mol

N is Avogadro's number (6.023×10^{23}/mol).

Dividing molecular weight M by the density ρ is M/ρ molar volume, and for solids, the additive property is generally applicable, which means it is the volume one mole of matter fills. The molar volume is as follows, since the comparison for packing factor V_i and atomic packing density V_t is also similar: Mole volume = M/ρ = V_i/V_t

That is, Vt equals $\rho(Vi/M)$. Actually, if glass of 30 mole percent Li_2O and 70 mole percent Si is examined you get the following. First, V_i of Li_2O and SiO_2 are calculated to be 8.51 and 14.0 cc/mol respectively. Therefore, V_t = (8.51 x 0.3 + 14.0 x 0.7) ρ/M = 12.353 ρ/M.

The molecular weight of this glass is 51.0, and with an actual density of ρ = 2.33, V_t = 0.564.

According to Makishima et al, this V_t is proportional to Young's modulus. Molecular weight is low following this formula, and moreover, Young's modulus becomes as high as that of high density glass.

Table 7-8 shows the specific gravity of experimental glasses and the value of V_t calculated from the specific gravity. The compressive strength is also noted. SAC-1 to SAC-7 on the table are glasses containing the Al_2O_3 - SiO_2 - CaF_2 three-dimensional system, and Figure 7-7 shows the V_t of these plotted on a triangular graph. By comparing this figure with Figure 7-2, it can be seen that composition with much Al_2O_3 have a high V_t and also a high compressive strength. Furthermore, examination of the values of V_t for the experimental glasses in Table 7-8 shows that the more Al_2O_3 in the glass, the more likely V_t will be high. The compressive strength and V_t also correspond well; compressive strength tends to be relatively large for the cement made from glass with a high V_t.

Since these values for compressive strength were obtained using laboratory methods, the values are much lower than those of commercial products due to the size of the powder particles being slightly larger. In other words, these figures are relative values rather than absolute values.

Compensation for the portion of the precipitated crystals was not done for the calculation of the atomic packing density. However, the atomic packing density of CaF_2 is about 0.605, and since there is not much difference with the atomic packing ratio of glass, the effect of the precipitated crystal was probably not that large. When the atomic packing ratio is 0.834 and α-Al_2O_3 precipitates, the effect may be large, but since the quantity of precipitate is extremely small compared to CaF_2, this may also not have much effect.

When the cut surface of hardened cement is observed with a scanning electron microscope, the craze lines are intragranular. Even from this viewpoint, it is easy to think that the strength of the core glass supports the strength of the set cement. That is, the matrix is a section useful in conducting external forces, and it is thought that the distortion, until the proportionality limit is reached, is quite large.

CHAPTER VIII
SUPPLEMENT

LIGHT-CURED
RESTORATIVE GLASS
IONOMER CEMENT

LIGHT-CURED RESTORATIVE GLASS IONOMER CEMENT

Shigeru Katsuyama and Isamu Nogami
Department of Operative Dentistry
Nippon Dental University

Kazuo Hirota
GC Corporation, Tokyo, Japan

Although glass ionomer cement has many distinctive features, its actual clinical use as a restorative material has been limited due to water sensitivity during initial setting, problems with transparency, and the cement's other disadvantages compared to composite resin. Improvement of the disadvantageous properties of the cement has been attempted through the use of light polymerization, a method of curing previously unavailable for glass ionomer cement. Light polymerization has been achieved by including a light polymerizing catalyst and monomer in the cement liquid.

By making the cement light curable, working time is increased so there is no hurry in placing the restoration. Further, water sensitivity is reduced by setting the cement by irradiation. The clinical procedures for placing restorations with light-curable glass ionomer cement are shown in Figure 8-1. Since a bonding agent is unnecessary, there are fewer clinical steps than for composite restorations. This may be particularly advantageous with pediatric patients.

The actual steps are as follows: after cavity preparation, the smear layer is removed with dentin conditioner; the shade of cement is selected after rinsing with water; the cement is mixed and placed; and visible light is used to set the material. After the glass ionomer has been set, it is adjusted and finished using a fine diamond bur, silicone points, and so on, avoiding contact with moisture. It is no longer necessary to wait between placement and finishing to prevent water sensitivity, as was required with previous types of glass ionomer cement restorations; this is a significant clinical improvement.

It is desirable to apply varnish to the surface after same-day finishing, since some chemical reaction will still be occurring. Varnishing enables the operator to produce a surface which is stable over the long term.

Distinctive Features

The distinctive features of light-cured glass ionomer cement can be summarized as follows.

1. Almost no water sensitivity after 20 seconds of irradiation.

Light curing makes it possible to finish the restoration under water irrigation. With the previous glass ionomer cements, it was necessary to wait about 20 minutes after placement when finishing was done on the same day. It is now possible to finish the cement immediately after light curing.

2. Shades harmonize well with tooth structure

The transparency of the hardened cement is greater than that of the former glasss ionomers, and esthetics are greatly improved. Because of this, the new material harmonizes well with natural tooth structure.

3. Early manifestation of properties

The basic properties of the cement appear quickly after setting, producing a stable condition. This is especially significant in actual clinical use. The physical properties of the

Figure 8-1. Comparison of clinical steps for light-cured glass ionomer cement and cnmposite restorations.

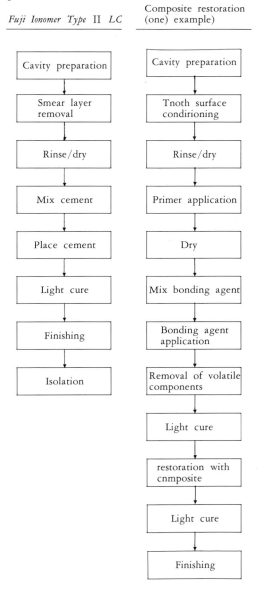

Fuji Ionomer Type II *LC*	Composite restoration (one) example
Cavity preparation	Cavity preparation
Smear layer removal	Tnoth surface condirioning
Rinse/dry	Rinse/dry
Mix cement	Primer application
Place cement	Dry
Light cure	Mix bonding agent
Finishing	Bonding agent application
Isolation	Removal of volatile components
	Light cure
	restoration with cnmposite
	Light cure
	Finishing

onds of exposure to light, all shades are set with certainty to a depth of 2.5 mm. Figure 8-3 shows changes in compressive strength over time for both the light-cured and the former types of cement. The light-cured type shows an extremely high compressive strength of 1800 kgf/cm² after just 10 minutes from the start of mixing (when light cured).

4. Superior biocompatibility

Biocompatibility, the most prominent feature of the former glass ionomer cements, is also not a problem with the new light-cured cements. This point was verified first with cell toxicity experiments and then with biological experiments.

5. Superior adhesion to both enamel and dentin

The light-cured glass ionomer shows greater adhesion to both enamel and dentin than the previous glass ionomers. Furthermore, its adhesion to tooth structure can be strengthened and also made more stable by removing the smear layer with GC *Dentin Conditioner*, as was also recommended for former glass ionomers.

6. Anticariogenic effect

The fluoride release of *Fuji II LC* over time is shown in Figure 8-4. The amount released initially is lower than that of the former type of glass ionomer, but both tend to release the same fixed quantity of fluoride over the long run.

7. Prognosis is easy to determine by radiopacity

Experiments to help broaden the clinical applications of light-cured glass ionomer cement's distinctive features of biocompatibility, adhesion to tooth structure, fluoride release, and esthetics will continue in the future, and as the properties of glass ionomer cements improve, another phase of development of this material can be expected.

cement are summarized in Table 8-1. The mechanical properties of the cement have been elevated compared to the previous glass ionomers, with tensile strength having been markedly increased, to twice that of the previous product.

The depth of polymerization from light curing is shown in Figure 8-2. After 20 sec-

Table 8-1. Physical properties of glass ionomer cement.

		Fuji Ionomer Type II LC	Fuji Ionomer Type II
Standard powder:liquid ratio (g/g)		3.0/1.0	2.7/1.0
Working time		3 min 15 sec	2min 00 sec
Setting time		light cure 20 sec	4 min 00 sec
Compressive strength at 24 hrs (kgf/cm²)		2180 (40)	2060 (120)
Tensile strength at 24 hours (kgf/cm²)		360 (40)	162 (22)
Bond strength at 24 hrs (kgf/cm²)	Bovine enamel	58 (10)	47 (8)
	Bovine dentin	53 (16)	44 (10)
Disintegration rate (%)	Pure water	0.07	0.07
	Lactic acid (0.001M)	0.25	0.33
Radiopacity		○	○

* ( ) is standard deviation

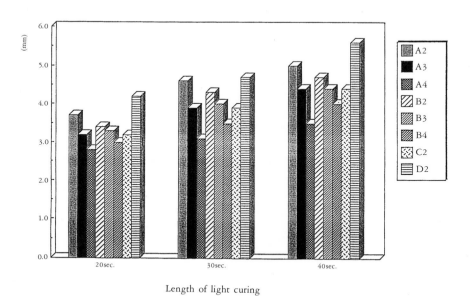

Length of light curing

Fig. 8-2. Curing depth of *Fuji Ionomer Type* II *LC.*

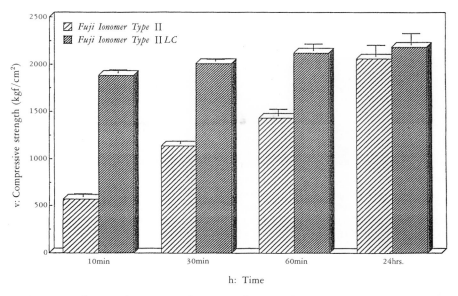

Fig. 8-3. Changes in compressive strength over time.

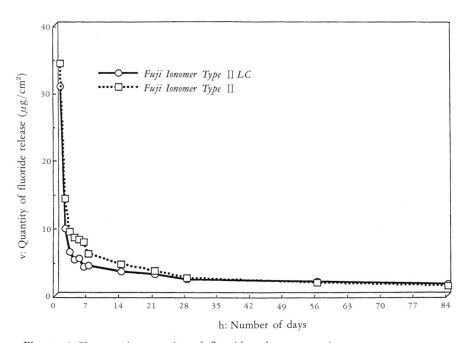

Fig. 8-4. Changes in quantity of fluoride release over time.

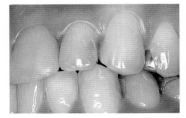

Fig. 8-5. Prior restoration. Maxillary left anterior teeth. Secondary caries can be seen on the distal of the maxillary left lateral incisor and surrounding the tooth-colored restoration. The caries on the distal surface are quite extensive, and unsupported enamel can be seen on the labial. A Class-III restoration has been planned for this lesion. The periodontal tissues are healthy.

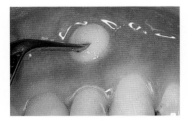

Fig. 8-6. Anesthetic. Anesthesia is achieved before beginning the procedure, if necessary. The area around the point of injection is disinfected and topical anesthetic is applied to the surface before administering the local anesthetic.

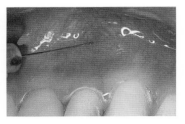

Fig. 8-7. Anesthetic. Anesthetic is injected through the point previously numbed with topical anesthetic.

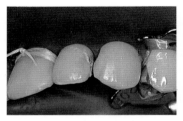

Fig. 8-8. Rubber dam isolation. The tooth is isolated with a rubber dam before cavity preparation. For restorative procedures, it is necessary to expose at a minimum both the proximal teeth for restorative procedures.

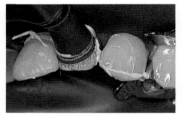

Fig. 8-9. Cleansing tooth surfaces. If there is stain from tobacco, food, or drink on the tooth where esthetic restorations are to be placed, the surface of the crown must always be cleansed using prophylaxis paste. If the cleansing is incomplete, accurate shade matching is difficult, and an esthetic restoration cannot be expected.

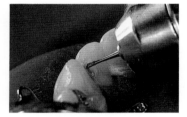

Fig. 8-10. Opening the cavity. Class III restorations on interproximal surfaces in anterior teeth must be started only after careful consideration of esthetic and technical aspects regarding whether to go in from the labial or lingual. In this case, the cavity was opened from the lingual because of esthetic considerations. When an existing restoration is removed before cavity preparation, it is probably best to use a small diameter bur or point (GC D-1) to preserve healthy tooth structure, and to also avoid injuring the adjacent teeth. When carbide burs are used, it is convenient to use carbide burs, such as pear-shaped burs (GC 330). (Mirror used.)

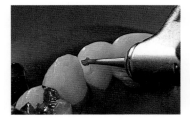

Fig. 8-11. Removal of soft dentin. Proceed in opening the cavity using round steel burs 006 to 016 (bur nos. 1/2-5). Healthy dentin is preserved as much as possible; the cavity outline is made as small as possible. Unsupported enamel is left in some cases. (Mirror used.)

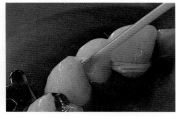

Fig. 8-12. Dying the soft dentin. If it is necessary, caries detection dye is used to make sure all the soft dentin is removed. (Mirror used.)

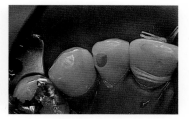

Fig. 8-13. Dying the soft dentin. The soft dentin and cutting debris from the bur have been dyed red in the cavity. The removal of soft dentin can be seen easily, especially at the point angles on both the labial and the lingual; care must be taken to completely remove the soft dentin since cases are frequently seen in which there is stain in these areas, creating severe problems for the prognosis of the tooth. It is necessary to confirm caries removal with a mirror in areas which cannot be seen directly. After that, the preparation is cleansed using oxydol, and then the cavity is rinsed again and dried. (Mirror used.)

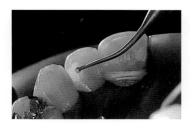

Fig. 8-14. Preparation completion, pulp capping. Cavity preparation has been completed. Since *Fuji 2 LC* adheres chemically to tooth structure, it is not necessary to provide special mechanical retention form. *Fuji 2 LC* is a restorative material which produces little stimulation of the dental pulp, so if the cavity is extremely deep and the remaining dentin is very thin, an indirect pulp cap of calcium hydroxide should be placed to protect the pulp. Care should be taken so as to not apply the calcium hydroxide on the enamel of the lateral walls to allow for maximum adhesion of the glass ionomer. But if the calcium hydroxide sticks to such areas, this excess capping material must be removed completely with a bur or hand instrument after it has hardened. (Mirror used.)

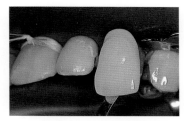

Fig. 8-15. Shade selection (*Vita Shade*). An appropriate shade of *Fuji 2 LC* is chosen by comparing the shade guide to the adjacent teeth. When natural lighting can be used, the shade should be chosen after the room illumination has been turned off. The shade is always chosen with the teeth in a moist state, using the central region of the shade guide. If it is difficult to select the shade using the *Vita shade guide*, an alternate method is to mix and cure a small piece of *Fuji 2 LC* and match it with the preparation.

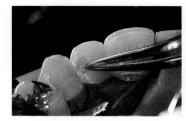

Fig. 8-16. Cleansing the preparation (GC Conditioner). Dentin conditioner is applied to the enamel at the cavity margin and to the dentin. Treatment time is approximately 20 to 30 seconds. Since the dentinal tubeless can be opened if dentin conditioner is applied for more than 30 seconds, long periods of treatment are avoided. (Mirror used.)

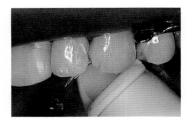

Fig. 8-17. Rinsing. 20 to 30 seconds after applying the conditioner, the preparation cavity is immediately rinsed with water for 20 seconds.

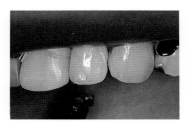

Fig. 8-18. Drying. The prepared cavity is adequately dried with oil-free air. It is important to see to it that the treatment surface is not soiled, but if by any chance it does become contaminated, the cleansing procedure is repeated, and the prepared cavity is then rinsed and dried again.

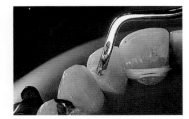

Fig. 8-19. Placing the glass ionomer cement (*Fuji 2 LC*). The *Fuji 2 LC* is carefully inserted into the prepared cavity, starting from at the line angles so as to not incorporate air bubbles. If the cavity is small, it is convenient to use a syringe. (Mirror used)

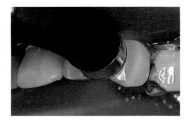

Fig. 8-20. Curing the glass ionomer cement (*Fuji 2 LC*). The restoration is light cured for a minimum of 20 seconds on both the labial and the lingual sides. The tip of the light is placed at right angles to the surface of the cavity, and the light is irradiated as close to the glass ionomer cement as possible. When there is no space between the strips, the surface is initially set with the first 2 to 3 seconds of the light a little away from the glass ionomer cement, and then the tip is placed on the surface so stability will be good. Since the strength of the light is inversely proportional to the square of the distance, the farther the tip of the light is separated from the glass ionomer cement, the worse the polymerization rate becomes. In case of large or deep cavity, the filling is divided into several increments, and a layered restoration is placed.

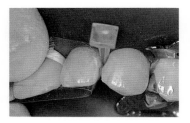

Fig. 8-21. Adjustment of the matrix. The adjusted and tried-in matrix is inserted between the teeth and is secured with a wedge.

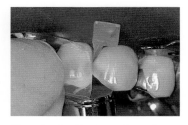

Fig. 8-22. Curing the glass ionomer cement (*Fuji 2 LC*). Light cure from both the labial and the lingual. A more complete set can be obtained by increasing the light curing time.

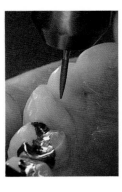

Fig. 8-23. Removal of excess cement. Excess cement at the line angles and on the labial is removed using *GC B-18ff*, and the anatomy is contoured at the same time. It is important to pay attention to details, not leaving a thin layer of excess cement or removing enamel. Adjustment and finishing are done in moist condition, but if the distinction between tooth structure and glass ionomer cement becomes difficult, enamel and glass ionomer cement can be easily distinguished finishing it dry, and shifting from restorative material to tooth structure can be easily done. (Mirror used.)

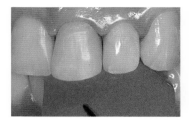

Fig. 8-24. Occlusal adjustment. Articulating paper should always be used to check the occlusion when lingual ridges are restored.

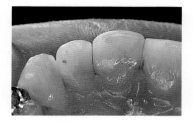

Fig. 8-25. Occlusal adjustment. High areas are removed with *GC C-17f*; not only centric occlusion, but also anterior movements should always be checked. (Mirror used.)

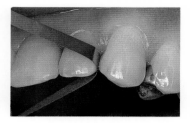

Fig. 8-26. Adjustment and polishing the proximal surface (*GC New Metal Strips*). Adjustment and polishing are all done in wet condition with the new GC metal strips. They are provided in four grits: #200, #300, #600, and #1000. It is important to always use them in the proper color-coded sequence of red, blue, green and then yellow. Anatomy can be modified effectively, but since the abrasive strength of the strips is also great, care must be taken so as to not loose the contact point, and in some cases, a separator should be used. Also, three types of widths are available: A 2.6 mm, B 3.3 mm, C 4.0 mm, so whichever is needed for each case can be used.

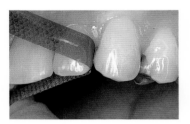

Fig. 8-27. Epitex finishing strips are used to polish the proximal surface. These come in 4 grits: blue (coarse), green (medium), gray (fine), and pink (extra fine), and by using them one after the other, a smooth, polished surface can be obtained.

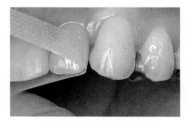

Fig. 8-28. Polishing the proximal surface (*Epitex*). With a thickness of 0.05 mm, insertion of the finishing strips even into tight contacts goes smoothly, and care must be taken not to lose the contact. A separator is used in some cases, and the strips are used in sequence, starting with the dark color.

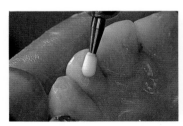

Fig. 8-29. Polishing (*GC White Alundum Points*). White alundum points are used to polish the lingual surface in a moist condition. (Mirror used.)

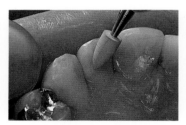

Fig. 8-30. Polishing (*GC Micro gray silicone points*). The final polishing on the lingual surface is completed using Micro-gray silicone points. If excessive pressure is applied, heat will be generated and craze lines will appear on the surface of glass ionomer cement. So polishing must be done carefully. (Mirror used.)

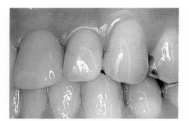

Fig. 8-31. Completed restoration. Restoration of the complex cavity on the left distal surface completed.

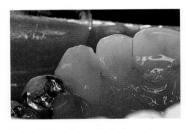 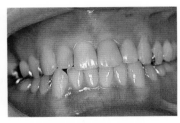

Fig. 8-32. Completed restoration. View from the lingual. (Mirror used.)

Fig. 8-33. Completed restoration. View of the entire anterior region.

Fuji II LC Clinical Manual
Tooth Nos. 23, 24, 25
Wedge Shape Defect

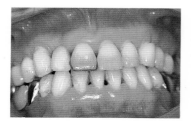

Fig. 8-34. Prior restoration. The entire anterior region. Toothbrush abrasion can be seen on the maxillary left central incisor back to the second premolar extending from the cervical region onto the root surface.

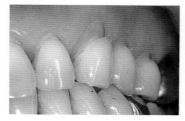

Fig. 8-35. Prior restoration. The upper left maxillary region has been enlarged. The lesions from the canine to the second premolar are particularly deep, approaching the dental pulp, and the patient complains of pain from stimulation by cold water, etc. Surrounding gingiva are healthy.

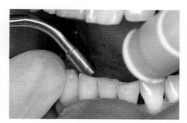

Fig. 8-36. Cleansing the tooth surface. When placing esthetic restorations, the surface of the crown must be cleansed if there is tobacco stain on the tooth surface. Simple removal is possible by using the air flow syringe.

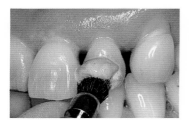

Fig. 8-37. Cleansing the tooth surface. The surface of the crown is cleansed using prophylaxis paste and a rubber cup. Accurate shade selection is difficult if cleansing is incomplete, and an esthetic restoration cannot be expected.

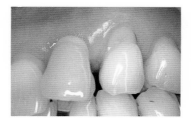

Fig. 8-38. Shade selection (*Vita shade*). The appropriate shade of *Fuji 2 LC* is selected by comparing the shade guide to the adjacent teeth. When natural light can be used, the room lights are turned off and the shade is selected. When it is difficult to select a shade with the Vita shade guide, an alternate method is to mix some *Fuji 2 LC*, cure a small piece and match it to the cavity. Shade selection is always done with teeth in a moist condition.

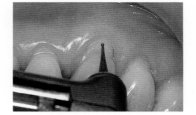

Fig. 8-39. Preparation completion. The cavity wall is formed with a round bur following the outline of the wedge-shaped lesion, and the preparation is completed. Since *Fuji 2 LC* chemically adheres to tooth structure, it is not necessary to provide special mechanical retention form. *Fuji 2 LC* is a restorative material which produces little stimulation of the dental pulp. If the cavity is extremely deep and the remaining dentin is very thin, an indirect pulp cap of calcium hydroxide should be placed in the cavity to protect the pulp.

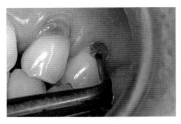

Fig. 8-40. Cleansing the preparation (*GC Dentin Conditioner*) Dentin conditioner is applied to the enamel at the cavity margin and to the dentin. Treatment time is approximately 20 to 30 seconds. Since the dentinal tubules can be opened if dentin conditioner is applied for more than 30 seconds, long treatment times are avoided.

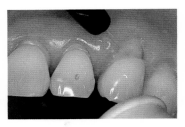

Fig. 8-41. Rinsing. 20 to 30 seconds after applying the conditioner, the prepared cavity is immediately rinsed with water for 20 or more seconds.

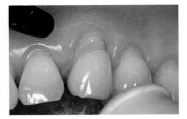

Fig. 8-42. Drying. The prepared cavity is dried adequately with oil free air. It is necessary to be careful that the treated surface is not soiled, but if by any chance it does become contaminated, the cleansing treatment is repeated, and the preparation is then rinsed and dried.

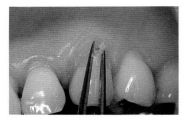

Fig. 8-43. Matrix try-in (*Hawe Cervial Matrices, transparent*). A matrix which is light-permeable and fits the curvature of the cervical region of the tooth is chosen.

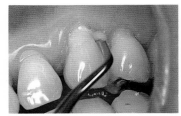

Fig. 8-44. Placing the glass ionomer cement (*Fuji 2 LC*). *Fuji 2 LC* is carefully inserted into the prepared cavity starting from at the line angles so as to not incorporated air bubbles. If the cavity is small, it is convenient to use a syringe. When the prepared cavity is large or deep, the limitations concerning polymerization shrinkage and setting must be considered, and the glass ionomer is divided into several portions and placed incrementally.

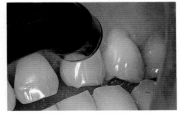

Fig. 8-45. Curing the (*GC VL2*) glass ionomer cement (*Fuji 2 LC*). The glass ionomer cement is cured for a minimum of 20 seconds. The tip of the light is placed at right angles to the surface of the cavity, and is irradiated as close to the glass ionomer cement as possible. When there is no space between the strips or matrix the surface is initially set with the first 2 to 3 seconds irradiation a little away from the glass ionomer cement, and then the tip is placed on the surface, so the stability will be good. Since the strength of the light is inversely proportional to the square of the distance, the farther the tip of the light is separated from the glass ionomer cement, the worse the polymerization becomes.

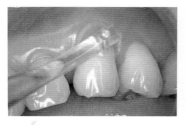

Fig. 8-46. Pressure from the matrix. The preparation cavity is filled with *Fuji 2 LC*, and pressure is carefully applied to the cement using the matrix so that air bubbles will not incorporated.

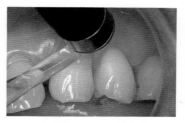

Fig. 8-47. Curing the glass ionomer cement (*Fuji 2 LC*). Using a visible curing light (*GC VL 2*), the light is irradiated at right angles to the cavity surface. A more complete set can be obtained by increasing the light curing time, but it is not the case that the longer the cure, the better. For example, if the length of light curing is complete, but some part is still inadequate, there should be no cause to worry because that portion will polymerizes chemically.

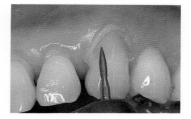

Fig. 8-48. Removal of excess. The excess on the labial is removed using *GC B-18ff* and the anatomy is contoured at the same time. It is important to pay attention to details, either leaving a thin layer of excess cement nor removing enamel. Adjustment and finishing are done in moist condition if the distinction between tooth structure and glass ionomer cement becomes difficult, enamel and glass ionomer cement can be easily distinguished if finishing is done dry, and shifting from the restorative material toward the tooth structure can be done easily.

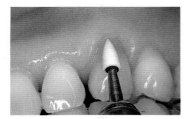

Fig. 8-49. Polishing (*GC White Alundum Points*). Polishing the flat surfaces should be always done in moist condition, white alundum points. Since the compressive strength after 10 seconds irradiation curing reaches approximately 80% of that after 24 hours, it is possible to start polishing immediately, but the results produced by polishing after 24 hours are even better.

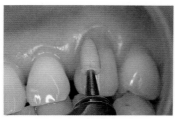

Fig. 8-50. Polishing (*GC Micro Gray Silicone Points*). Final polishing of the flat surfaces is completed using micro gray silicone points. If excessive pressure is applied, heat will be generated, and craze lines will appear on the surface of the glass ionomer cement, so polishing must be done carefully under moist conditions, without too much pressure.

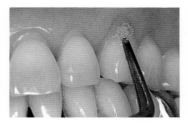

Fig. 8-51. Application of varnish (*Fuji Varnish*). Since the chemical polymerization reaction continues even after same day finishing, it is desirable to apply varnish to the surface after finishing. A long term stable surface will be obtained.

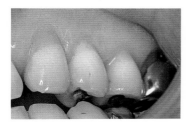

Fig. 8-52. Treatment completed. Restoration of the wedge shape defect lesions have been completed.

R E F E R E N C E S

A. History·Total Estimation

A1 Smith, D.C.: A new dental cement, Br. Dent. J. 125: 381–384, 1968.

A2 Wilson, A.D., and Kent, B.E.: A new translucent cement for dentistry, The glass ionomer cement, Br. Dent. J. 132(2): 133–135, 1972.

A3 Kawahara, H. et al.: The application of glass-ionomer cement to dentistry, Dent. Outlook 50(4): 623–633, 1977. (Japanese)

A4 Tani, Y., and Ida, K.: Study on ASPA cement, Int. J. Dent. Med. 6(2): 159–166, 1977. (Japanese)

A5 Ida, K., and Tani, Y.: Study on dental restorative materials glass Ionomer cement, Int. J. Dent. Med. 6(3): 303–308, 1977. (Japanese)

A6 Kawahara, H. et al.: The application of fuji glass-ionomer cement to dentistry, Int. J. Dent. Med. 6(4): 479–480, 1977. (Japanese)

A7 Saito, S., and Tomita, K.: Study on glass-ionomer cement, Dent. Diamond 2(12): 78–81, 1977. (Japanese)

A8 Hirasawa, T.: Chemistry of dental materials. (1) Dental cements based on polycarboxylic acid, Tsurumi Univ. Dent. J. 3(1): 9–13, 1977. (Japanese)

A9 Wilson, A.D.: The development of glass-ionomer cements, Dent. update. Oct: 401–412, 1977.

A10 McLean, J.W., and Wilson, A.D.: The clinical development of the glass-ionomer cement. II. Some clinical applications, Aust. Dent. J. 22(31): 120–127, 1977.

A11 Sato, S. et al.: Study on glass-ionomer cement. (3) Luting property, J.J. Res. Sci. Dent. Mater. Appli. 35(1): 68–79, 1978. (Japanese)

A12 Masaka, N. et al.: The latest trend of new dental restorative materials. Part 1 Characteristic of dental cements and how to use, Dent. Outlook 52(4): 663–674, 1978 (Japanese)

A13 Tomioka, K.: Composite materials and glass-ionomer, Dent. Diamond 3(11): 44–47, 1978. (Japanese)

A14 Saito, S.: The nature of the glass-ionomer cement, J. Dent. Med. 10; 104–125, 1979. (Japanese)

A15 Onose, H.: Study on dental restorative glass-ionomer cement, J. Tokyo Dent. Ass. 27(3): 2–9, 1979. (Japanese)

A16 Kondo, S. et al.: Study on luting cements. Part 3, J. Hokkaido Dent. Ass. 34: 135–141, 1979. (Japanese)

A17 McLean, J.W.: The future of restorative materials, J. of prosthet. Dent. 42: 154–158, 1979.

A18 Tomioka, K.: Study on glass-ionomer cement, Dent. Diamond 5(9): 26–28, 1980. (Japanese)

A19 Saito, S.: Luting and filling cements. GC fuji ionomer, J. Dent. Enginee. 54: 14–15, 1980. (Japanese)

A20 Saito, A.: Requirement of clinical demand and material, Dent. Diamond 5(3): 78–81, 1980. (Japanese)

A21 Ishikawa, T.: Characteristic of glass-ionomer cement & uses. J. Tokyo Dent. Ass. 31(9): 11–17, 1983. (Japanese)

A22 The application of glass-ionomer cement to clinic. Dent. Diamond 8(2): 38–39, 1983. (Japanese)

A23 Horn, H.R.: The current status of dental luting cements, N.S.Y. Dent. J. Oct: 549–551, 1983.

A24 Hara, G.: Treatment of dental caries. (I) Disease of the hard tissues. Glass-ionomer cement, Dent. Outlook 63(2): 377–383, 1984. (Japanese)

A25 Hashimoto, K. et al.: How to use for luting materials, J. Dent. Enginee. 70: 1–13, 1984. (Japanese)

A26 McLean, J.W. et al.: Development and use of water-hardening glass ionomer luting cements, J. Prosthet. Dent. 52(2): 175, 1984.

A27 Ishida, K. et al.: Plastic-filling materials 3 glass-ionomer cement, Dent. Information 49(3): 21–25, 1985. (Japanese)

A28 Atkinson, A.S., and Pearson, G.J.: The evolution of glass-ionomer cements, Br. Dent. J. 159(10): 335–337, 1985.

A29 Benji, F.: The history and characteristic of glass-ionomer cement, J. P.F.A. 21: 29–45, 1986. (Japanese)

A30 Takigawa, T. et al.: Clinical evaluation of new luting glass-ionomer cement "New fuji ionomer", Nihon Univ. Dent. J. 61(1): 96–98, 1986. (Japanese)

A31 Walls, A.W.G.: Glass polyalkenoate (glass-ionomer) cements. A review, J. Dent. 14: 231–246, 1986.

A32 Knibbs, P.J. *et al.*: The performance of a zinc polycarboxylate luting cement and a glass-ionomer luting cement in general dental practice, Br. Dent. J. Jan: (11): 13–15, 1986.

A33 Knibbs, P.J. *et al.*: An evaluation of an anhyclrous glass-ionomer cement in general dental practice, Br. Dent. J. Mar: (8): 170–172, 1986.

A34 Phillips, R.W.: Era of new biomaterials in esthetic dentistry, J.A.D.A. 115: 7E–12E (Special), 1987.

A35 Hasegawa, J.: Study on adhesive material and luting material-How to use and choice, Dent. Diamond 12(2): 14–29, 1987. (Japanese)

A36 Gerdts, G.J., and Murchison, D.F.: Clinical uses of glass ionomer cement. A literature review A. van de voorde, Quintessence Int. 19(1): 53–61, 1988.

A37 Swift, E.J. JR.: An update on glass ionomer cements, Quintessence Int. 19(2): 125–130, 1988.

A38 McLean, J.W.: Glass-ionomer cements, Br. Dent. J. 164(9): 293–300, 1988.

A39 Jendresen, N.D. *et al.*: Report of the committee on scientific investigation of the American Academy of restorative Dentistry, J. Prosthet. Dent. 59(6): 703–738, 1988.

A40 Wilson, A.D., and McLean, J.W.: Glass ionomer cement, 1st ed, 1988, Quintessence Publ. Co.

A41 Hickel, R., and Vob, A.: (Langzeit) erfahrungen mit glasionomerzementen, Dtsch. Zahnarztl. Z. 43(3): 263–271, 1988.

B. Composition·Hardening Reaction

B1 Wilson, A.D., and Kent, B.E.: Brit. Pat. application, No.61041/69, Br. Pat. 1316129, 1969.

B2 Crisp, S., and Wilson, A.D.: Reactions in glass ionomer cement. I. Decomposition of the powder, J. Dent. Res. 53(6): 1408–1413, 1974.

B3 Crisp, S. *et al.*: Reactions in glass ionomer cements. II. An infrared spectroscopic study, J. Dent. Res. 53(6): 1414–1419, 1974.

B4 Crisp, S., and Wilson, A.D.: Reactions in glass ionomer cements. III. The precipitation reaction, J. Dent. Res. 53(6): 1420–1424, 1974.

B5 Wilson, A.D., and Crisp, S.: Ionomer cement, Br. Polym. J. 7: 279–296, 1975.

B6 Crisp, S. *et al.*: Gelation of polyacrylic acid aqueous solutions and the measurement of viscosity, J. Dent. Res. 54(6): 1173–1175, 1975.

B7 Crisp, S. *et al.*: Zinc polycarboxylate cements. A chemical study of erosion and its relationship to molecular structure, J. Dent. Res. 55: 299–308, 1976.

B8 Crisp, S. *et al.*: An infra-red spectroscopic study of cement formation between mental oxides and aqueous solution of poly(acrylic acid), J. Mater. Sci. Letters. 36–48, 1976.

B9 Crisp, S., and Wilson, A.D.: Reactions in glass ionomer cements. V. Effect of incorporating tartaric acid in the cement liquid, J. Dent. Res. 55: 1023–1031, 1976.

B10 Crisp, S. *et al.*: Glass ionomer cements. Chemistry of erosion, J. Dent. Res. 55: 1032–1041, 1976.

B11 Crisp, S. *et al.*: Properties of improved glass-ionomer cement formulations, J. Dent. 3: 125–130, 1976.

B12 Hodd, K.A., and Reader, A.L.: The formation and hydrolytic stability of metal ion-polyacid gels, Br. Polym. J. Dec: 131–139, 1976.

B13 Wilson, A.D. *et al.*: Reactions in glass-ionomer cements. IV. Effect of chelating comonomers on setting behavior, J. Dent. Res. 55(3): 489–495, 1976.

B14 Crisp, S. *et al.*: Cement forming ability of silicate minerals and polyacid solution, J. Appl. Chem. Biotechnol. 27: 369–374, 1977.

B15 Wilson, A.D.: The chemistry of dental cements, Chem. Soc. Rev. 7: 265–296, 1978.

B16 Watts, D.C.: Cnmr spectroscopic analysis of poly(Electrolyte) cement liquids, J. Biomed. Mater. Res. 13: 423–435, 1979.

B17 Crisp, S. *et al.*: Characterization of glass-ionomer cements. 5. The effect of tartaric acid concentration in the liquid component, J. Dent. 7(4): 304–312, 1979.

B18 Kent, B.E. *et al.*: Glass ionomer cement formulations. I. The preparation of novel fluoroaluminosilicate glass high in fluorine, J. Dent. Res. 58(6): 1607–1619, 1979.

B19 Wilson, A.D. *et al.*: Aluminosilicate glasses for polyelectrolyte cements, Ind. Eng. Chem. Prod. Res. Dev. 19: 263–270, 1980.

B20 Crisp, S. *et al.*: Modification of ionomer cements by the addition of simple metal salts, Ind. Eng. Chem. Prod. Res. Dev. 19: 403–408, 1980.

B21 Crisp, S. *et al.*: Glass-ionomer cement formulations. II. The synthesis of novel polycarboxylic acids, J. Dent. Res. 59(6): 1055–1063, 1980.

B22 Lorton, L. *et al.*: Rheology of luting cements, J. Dent. Res. 59(9): 1486–1492, 1980.

B23 Prosser, H.J. *et al.*: NMR spectroscopy of dental materials. II. The role of tartaric acid in glass-ionomer cements, J. Biomed. Mater. Res. 16: 431–445, 1982.

B24 Prosser, H.J. *et al.*: The effect of additives on the setting properties of a glass-ionomer cement, J. Dent. Res. Oct: 1195–1198, 1982.

B25 Cook, W.D.: Setting of dental polyelectrolyte cements-viscosity studies of model systems, J. Biomed. Mater. Res. 17: 283–291, 1983.

B26 Cook, W.D.: Degrative analysis of glass ionomer polyelectrolyte cements, J. Biomed. Mater. Res. 17: 1015–1027, 1983.

B27 Yamamoto, Y.: The study on hydroxyapatite —Polyacrylic acid composite cement (Hidroxyapatite— Glass-ionomer cement), J.J. Dent. Mater 3(6): 787–796, 1984. (Japanese)

B28 McLean, J.W.: Alternatives to amalgam alloys. 1, Br. Dent. J. 157(2): 432–435, 1984.

B29 Prosser, H.J. *et al.*: Characterization of glass-ionomer cements 7. The physical properties of current materials, J. Dent. 12: 231–240, 1984.

B30 Lloyd, C.H.: A differential thermal analysis (DTA) for the heats of reaction and temperature rise produced during the setting of tooth coloured restorative materials, J. Oral Rehabil. 11: 111–121, 1984.

B31 Hill, R.G., and Wilson, A.D.: A rheological study of the role of additives on the setting of glass-ionomer cements, J. Dent. Res. 67(12): 1446–1450, 1988.

B32 Fusayama, T.: New dental cements, 1972, Nagasue Shoten. (Japanese)

B33 Hosoda, H. *et al.*: Part 1. The cored structure of three luting cements obtained by using Cryo-SEM and image analyzer, J.J. Dent. Mater. Dev. 9: 197–204, 1990. (Japanese)

B34 Wakumoto, S.: Operative dentistry, 1980, Ishiyaku Publishers, Inc. (Japanese)

B35 Maeda, T. *et al.*: unpublished.

B36 Ogata, N. *et al.*: Studies on glass-ionomer cement —Relationship between chemical composition of powders and compressive strength—, J.J. Conserv. Dent. 34: 209–227, 1991. (Japanese)

B37 Maeda, T. *et al.*: Studies on glass-poly (alkenoate) cement —Identity and morphology of crystallite in culsium fluoroalumino silicate glasses—, J.J. Conserv. Dent. 35: 482–488, 1992. (Japanese)

B38 Lowenstein, K.L.: Studies in the composition and structure of glasses possessing high Young's moduli, Part 1, The composition of high Young' modulus glasses and the function of individual ion in the glass structure, Phys. Chem. Glasses. 2: 69–82, 1961.

B39 Makishima, A., and Mackenzie, J.D.: Direct calculation of Young's modulus of glass, J. Non-crystalline Solids. 12: 35–45, 1973.

B40 Makishima, A., and Mackenzie, J.D.: Calculation of bulk modulus, shear modulus and poisson's ratio of glass, J. Non-Crystalline Solids. 17: 147–157, 1975.

B41 Anderson, O.L., and Nafe, J.E.: The bulk modulus—volume relationship for oxide compounds and related geophysical problem, J. Geophys. Res. 70: 3951–3963, 1965.

B42 Soga, N., and Anderson, O.L.: Comparison of elastic moduli between the glassy and crystalline state. Reprinted from VII International congress, on glass proceedings, Vol. 1 Science and Technology Article. 37: 1–9, 1966. Lamont Geological Observatory, Columbia Univ. Palisades, New York.

B43 Bridge, B., and Higazy, A.A.: A model of the compositional dependence of the elastic moduli of polycomponent oxide glasses, Phys. Chem. Glasses. 27: 1–14, 1986.

C. Physical Properties

C1 Kent, B.E. *et al.*: The properties of a glass ionomer cement, Br. Dent. J. 135(6): 322–326, 1973.

C2 Tomioka, K., and Saito, S.: Study on dental material science. (12) Filling material Part 3 glass-ionomer cement, Dent. Diamond 2(12): 78–81, 1977. (Japanese)

C3 Arai, K. *et al.*: Study on adhesive materials for restoration. (6) Physical, Bull. Josai Dent. Univ. 6(1): 173–179, 1977. (Japanese)

C4 McLean, J.W., and Wilson, A.D.: The clinical development of the glass-ionomer cement. I. Formulations and properties, Aust. Dent. J. 22(1): 31–36, 1977.

C5 McLean, J.W., and Wilson, A.D.: The clinical development of the glass-ionomer cement. III. The erosion lesion, Aust. Dent. J. 22(3): 190–195, 1977.

C6 Maldonado, A. *et al.*: An *in vitro* study of certain properties of a glass ionomer cement, J.A.D.A. 96(May): 785–792, 1978.

C7 Lorton, L. *et al.*: Measuring the apparent viscosity of dental cements, Dental Materials Group AADR/IADR. Abstract. No.213, 1978.

C8 Irie, M. *et al.*: Study on glass-ionomer-cement (3) Luting property, J.J. Dent. Mater. 36(2): 259, 1979. (Japanese)

C9 Tomigaya, J. *et al.*: Study on finishing and polishing of glass-ionomer cement, J.J. Conserv. Dent. 22(3): 414–424, 1979. (Japanese)

C10 Saito, S.: Dental esthetic restoration materials (Part 4), Dent. Diamond 4(8): 69–72, 1979. (Japanese)

C11 Jones, D.W. *et al.*: Direct tensile strength of glass ionomer, polycarboxylate and phosphate cements, J. Dent. Res. 57(394): Spec. Abst. 1212, 1979.

C12 McCabe, J..F. *et al.*: Some properties of a glass ionomer cement, Br. Dent. J. 146(9): 279–281, 1979.

C13 Crisp, S. *et al.*: The quantitative measurement of the opacity of anesthetic dental filling materials, J. Dent. Res. 58(6): 1585–1596, 1979.

C14 Wilson, A.D. *et al.*: The hydration of dental cements, J. Dent. Res. 58(3): 1065–1071, 1979.

C15 Irie, M.: Study on glass-ionomer cement (5) New luting glass-ionomer cement, J.J. Dent. Mater. 38(2): 8, 1981. (Japanese)

C16 Welker, V.D.: Aluminium-sililko-polyakrylatzement(ASPA)im vergleichendwerksto ffkundlichen test, Dtsch. Zahnarztl. Z. 36(8): 478–487, 1981.

C17 Tay, W.M., and Braden, M.: Dielectric properties of glass ionomer cements, J. Dent. Mater. 60(7): 1311–1314, 1981.

C18 Watts, D.C., and Smith, R.: Thermal diffusivity in finite cylindrical specimens of dental cements, J. Dent. Res. 60(12): 1972–1976, 1981.

C19 Irie, M. *et al.*: J.J. Dent. Mater. 38(4): 647–657, 1982. (Japanese)

C20 Irie, M. *et al.*: Study on glass-ionomer-cement (7) Study on characteristic change in relation to the passage of time, Part 2, J.J. Res. Sci. Dent. Mater. Appli. 1(4): 428, 1982. (Japanese)

C21 Takigawa, T.: Study on glass-ionomer cement, Influence of powder, J.J. Conserv. Dent. 25(3): 812–813, 1982. (Japanese)

C22 Cook, W.D.: Dental polyelectrolyte cements I. Biomaterials. 3(Oct): 232–236, 1982.

C23 Hirano, Y.: Study on characteristic changes in glass-ionomer cement for luting, in Relation to the passage of time, J.J. Dent. Mater. Dev. 2(6): 820–823, 1983. (Japanese)

C24 Irie, M. *et al.*: Change in physical properties of glass ionomer cements for luting following immersion in water up to 12 months, J.J. Dent. Mater. Dev. 2(6): 820–823, 1983. (Japanese)

C25 Yamaga, R. *et al.*: Physical properties of HY bond glass ionomer cement, Quintessence 7(2): 59–69, 1983. (Japanese)

C26 Cook, W.D.: Dental polyelectrolyte cements II. Biomaterials. 4(Jan): 21–24, 1983.

C27 Cook, W.D.: Dental polyelectrolyte cements III. Biomaterials. 4(Apl.): 85–88, 1983.

C28 Asmussen, E.: Opacity of glass-ionomer cements, Acta. Odontol. Scand. 41: 155–157, 1983.

C29 Yamamoto, Y.: An *in vitro* study on the reminerlizatio of inner carious dentin. Tsurumi Univ. Dent. J. 10(1): 57–74, 1984. (Japanese)

C30 Hashimoto, K., and Tawaragi, T.: A characteristic for glass-ionomer cement, Dent. Diamond 9(14): 50–55, 1984. (Japanese)

C31 Sugawara A. *et al.*: Change color of dental esthetic restorative materials, J. Tokyo Dent. Ass. 32(8): 278–286, 1984. (Japanese)

C32 Wilson, A.D., and Prosser, H.J.: A survey of inorganic and polyelectrolyte cements, Br. Dent. J. 157(12): 449–454, 1984.

C33 Lloyd, C.H.: A differential thermal analysis (DTA) for the heats of reaction, J. Oral. Rehabil. 11: 111–121, 1984.

C34 McLean, J.W. *et al.*: Development and use of water-hardening glass-ionomer luting cements, J. Prosthet. Dent. 52(2): 175–181, 1984.

C35 Tay, W.M., and Braden, M.: Dielectric properties of glass ionomer cements—further studies, J. Dent. Res. 63(1): 74–75, 1984.

C36 Formation and compressive strength of the ionomer cements prepar, J. Mater. Sci. Letters. 617–619, 1984.

C37 Marolf, R.: Glasionomerzemente-Materialeigenschaften und klinische anwendungeitve literatubersicht, Schweiz. Mschr. Zahnmed. 94(2): 117–133, 1984.

C38 Dag Brune, Dag Magnar Evje: Initial acidity of dental cements, Scand. J. Dent. Res. 92: 156–160, 1984.

C39 Watts, D.C. and Smith, R.: Thermal diffusion in some polyelectrolyte dental cements. The effect of powder/liquid ratio, J. Oral Rehabil. 11: 285–288, 1984.

C40 Sakamoto, Y. *et al.*: Study on glass-ionomer cement influence of elution and surface hardening of hardened material in the acid solution as priticle grain size of atomization, Nihon Univ. Dent. J. 59: 1, 129, 1985. (Japanese)

C41 Ishida, H. *et al.*: Plastic filling materials (3) Glass-ionomer cement, Dent. Information 49(3): 21–25, 1985. (Japanese)

C42 Phillips, S., and Bishop, B.M.: An *in vitro* study of the effect of moisture on glass-ionomer cement, Quintessence Int. 2: 175–177, 1985.

C43 Solomon, A., and Beech, D.R.: Bonding of composite to dentin using primers, Dent. Mater. 1: 79–82, 1985.

C44 Kanie, T.: Dimensional changes of luting cements after setting, Dent. Mater. J. 4(1): 40–46, 1985.

C45 Golden, M.: Fracture properties of composite and glass ionomer dental restorative materials, J. Biomed. Mater. Res. 19: 771–783, 1985.

C46 Yoshida, T. *et al.*: Experiment of glass-ionomer cement, Dent. Engee. 79: 18–28, 1989. (Japanese)

C47 Sakamoto, Y.: Study of glass-ionomer cement. Effect of the small particle size of powder on the physical properties, J.J. Conserv. Dent. 29(1): 95–105, 1986. (Japanese)

C48 Sakamoto, Y. *et al.*: Study on glass-ionomer cement. Influence of powder's atomization for interlocking force of underwater's cement, J.J. Conserv. Dent. 29(1): 500, 1986. (Japanese)

C49 Yasuda, A.: The influence of decomposition and salivas PH for glass-ionomer cement, J. Tokyo Dent. Coll. Soci. 74(4): 858–873, 1986. (Japanese)

C50 Oilo, G., and Evje, D.M.: Film thickness of dental luting cements. dental materials, Dent. Mater. 2: 85–89, 1986.

C51 Kullman, W.: Glasionomer-zemente-physikalischtechnische eigenschaften in abhängigkeit von der verarbeitung, Dtsch. Zahnarztl. Z. 41(8): 751–754, 1986.

C52 Mccullock, A.J., and Smith, B.G.N.: *In vitro* studies of cuspal movement produced by adhesive restorative materials, Br. Dent. J. 161(11): 405–409, 1986.

C53 Mount, G.J.: Longevity of glass ionomer cements, J. Prosthet. Dent. 55(6): 682–685, 1986.

C54 Physical property of glass ionomer cement, J.J. Dent. Ass. 40(2): 167–181, 1987.

C55 Ando, S.: Study on glass ionomer cement, J.J. Conserv. Dent. 30(5): 1987. (Japanese)

C56 Sinkai, K. *et al.*: A study on toothbrush abrasion of the restorative materials. Part I, Influence of the apparatus condition abrasion. J.J.

Conserv. Dent. 30(4): 1235–1244, 1987. (Japanese)

C57 Van Dijken, J.W.V., and Horstedt, P.: Effects of 5% sodium hypochlorite or tubulicid pretreatment *in vivo* on the marginal adaptation of dental adhesives and glass ionomer cements. Dent. Mater. 3(6): 303–306, 1987.

C58 Tay, W.M., and Braden, M.: Thermal diffusivity of glass-ionomer cements, J. Dent. Res. 66(5): 1040–1043, 1987.

C59 McKinney, J.E. *et al.*: Wear and microhardness of glass-ionomer cements, J. Dent. Res. 66(6): 1134–1139, 1987.

C60 Mechanism for erosion of glass ionomer cement in an acidic buffer solution, J. Dent. Res. 66(12): 1770–1774, 1987.

C61 Walls, A.W.G. *et al.*: The properties of glass polyalkenoate (Ionomer) cement incorporating sintered metallic particles, Dent. Mater. 3(3): 113–116, 1987.

C62 Mccabe, J.F., and Ogden, A.R.: The relationship between porosity, Compressive fatigue limit and wear in composite resin restorative materials, Dent. Mater. 3: 9–12, 1987.

C63 Yoshikawa, H.: Study on glass ionomer cement. Nihon Univ. Dent. J. 62(1): 44–55, 1988.

C64 Irie, M.: The applications and characteristics of glass ionomer cement to dentistry. Glass ionomer. Adhesive property. Physical property. Size change. Marginal shut, J. Tokyo Dent. Ass. 6(4): 257–261, 1988. (Japanese)

C65 Kanie, T. *et al.*: Studies on dental cements. Part 2. Dimensional changes of luting cements during setting, J.J. Conserv. Dent. 31(2): 324–331, 1988. (Japanese)

C66 Watanabe, H. *et al.*: A study on toothbrush abrasion of restorative materials, J.J. Conserv. Dent. 31(3): 775–781, 1988. (Japanese)

C67 Feilzer, A.J. *et al.*: Curing contraction of composites and glass-ionomer cements, J. Prothet. Dent. 59(3): 297–300, 1988.

C68 Omar, R.: A comparative study of the retentive capacity of dental cementing agents, J. Prosthet. Dent. 60(1): 35–40, 1988.

C69 Kullmann, W.: Die glaspolyalkenoat-kunststoff-füllung, Dtsch. Zahnarztl. Z. 43(3): 387–389, 1988.

C70 Hill, R.G., and Wilson, A.D.: Rheological study of the role of additives on the setting of glass-ionomer cements, J. Dent. Res. 67(12): 1446–1450, 1988.

C71 Kullmann, W.: Unersuchungen zur bearbeitungsfäehigkeit von aufbauwerk-stoffen auf polyelektrolytbasis, Dtsch. Zahnarztl. Z. 43(8): 843–846, 1988.

C72 Kullman, W.: Schleif- und polierpasten zur oberfläechenbearbeitung von kompositkunst-stoffen und glaspolyalkenoat-zementen, Dtsch. Zahnarztl. Z. 43(8): 923–928, 1988.

D. Adhesive Property

D1 Uetani, I.: Study on the filling cement for adhesion, J.J. Res. Sci. Dent. Mater. Appli. 33(3): 213–230, 1976. (Japanese)

D2 Hotz, P. et al.: The bonding of glass ionomer cements to metal and tooth substrates, Br. Dent. J. 142: 41–47, 1977.

D3 Prodger, T.E., and Symonds, M.: ASPA adhesion study, Br. Dent. J. 143(8): 266–270, 1977.

D4 Levine, R.S. et al.: Improving the bond strength of polyacrylate cements to dentine, Br. Dent. J., 143:8, 275–277, 1977.

D5 Vougiouklakis, G., and Smith, D.C.: Bonding of restorative materials to teeth, J. Dent. Res. 57: 340–, 1978.

D6 Hayakawa, T.: The effect of surface coarse for luting cements and bonding strength, J. Tokyo Dent. Coll. Soc. 67(2): 290–301, 1979. (Japanese)

D7 Yedid, S.E., and Kai Chiu Chan: Bond strength of three esthetic restorative materials to enamel and dentin, J. Prosthet. Dent. 44(5): 573–576, 1980.

D8 Goto, T.: Retention efficiency of three luting cements, J.J. Dent. App. Mater. 22(59): 168–171, 1981. (Japanese)

D9 Negm, M.M. et al.: An evaluation of mechanical and adhesive properties of poly-carboxylate and glass ionomer cements, J. Oral. Rehabil. 9: 161–167, 1982.

D10 Powis, D.R. et al.: Improved adhesion of a glass ionomer cement to dentin and enamel, J. Dent. Res. 61(12): 1416–1422, 1982.

D11 Coury, T.L. et al.: Adhesiveness of glass-ionomer cement to enamel and dentin. A laboratory study, Oper. Dent. 7: 2–6, 1982.

D12 Wilson, A.D. et al.: Mechanism of adhesion of polyelectrolyte cements to hydroxyapatite, J. Dent. Res. 62(5): 590–592, 1983.

D13 Ray, N.J.: Aspects of adhesion in dentistry-Part I. The traditional restorative materials: zinc phosphate, silver amalgam and the sili-cates, J. Irish Dent. Assoc. May-June: 31–34, 1983.

D14 Ray, N.J.: Aspects of adhesion in dentistry-Part II. Polycarboxylates and glass ionomers, J. Irish Dent. Assoc. May-June: 35–39, 1983.

D15 Watts, T.L.P. et al.: Initial physical tests of aluminoborate cements in the context of periodontal dressing development, J. Oral Rehabil. 10: 393–398, 1983.

D16 Inoue, Y. et al.: The adhesive property of organic cement to tooth structure Part 1. The adhesive property of glass ionomer cement to dentin treated with various condi-tioners, J.J. Dent. Mater. Dev. 3(5) 696–701, 1984. (Japanese)

D17 Richter, W.A., and Macentee, M.I.: The effect of a microbicidal cleaner on the retentive strength of two cements, J. Prosthet. Dent. 51(1): 46–48, 1984.

D18 Beech, D.R. et al.: Bond strength of polycarboxylic acid cements to treated den-tine, Dent. Mater. 1: 154–157, 1985.

D19 Tyas, M.J., and Beech, D.R.: Clinical perfor-mance of three restorative materials for non-undercut cervical abrasion resins, Aust. Dent. J. 30(4): 260–264, 1985.

D20 Lacefield, W.R. et al.: Tensile bond strength of a glass-ionomer cement, J. Prosthet. Dent. 53(2): 194–198, 1985.

D21 Dilts, W.E. et al.: Relative shear bond strengths of luting media with various core materials, J. Prosthet. Dent. 53(4): 505–508, 1985.

D22 Tohno, N.: The adhesive properties of glass-ionomer cement to substance, J.J. Dent. Ass. 49(6) 856–857, 1986. (Japanese)

D23 Gordon, A.A. et al.: Bond strength of com-posite to composite and bond strength of composite to glass ionomer lining cements, General Dent. July-August: 290–293, 1986.

D24 Aboush, Y.E.Y., and Jenkins, C.B.G.: An evaluation of the bonding of glass-ionomer restoratives to dentine and enamel, Br. Dent. J. 161(6): 179–184, 1986.

D25 Tyas, M.J. et al.: Clinical evaluation of scotchbond, one year results, Aust. Dent. J. 31(3): 159–164, 1986.

D26 Hinoura, K. et al.: Influence of dentine sur-face treatments on the bond strengths of dentin-lining cements, Oper. Dent. 11: 147–154, 1986.

D27 Barakat, M.M., and Powers, J.M.: In vitro bond strength of cements to treated teeth, Aust. Dent. J. 31: 415, 1986.

D28 Nasu, T.: Polyacrylic acid-metal adhesive bond joint characterization by oyphoto electron spectroscopy, J. Biomed. Mater. Res. 20: 347–362, 1986.

D29 Tohno, N.: Bond characteristics of a glass-ionomer cement to human tooth, J.J. Dent. App. Mater. 6:(4) 449–464, 1987. (Japanese)

D30 Tjan, A.H.L. *et al.*: Effects of various cementation methods on the retention of prefabricated posts, J. Prosthet. Dent. 58(3): 309–313, 1987.

D31 Irie, M., and Nakai, H.: The marginal gap and bonding strength of glass ionomers, Dent. Mater. 6(1): 46–53, 1987.

D32 Kitano, T.: Tensil bond strength of adhesive cements to base cements and core materials, J.J. Dent. App. Mater. 7(3): 488–502, 1988. (Japanese)

D33 Jaijer, R., and Smith, D.C.: A comparison between zinc phosphate and glass ionomer cement in orthodontics, American J. Orthod. Dentofac. Orthop. 93(4): 273–279, 1988.

D34 Oilo, G., and Evje, D.M.: A bend test for measuring cement-dentin bond, Dent. Mater. 4: 98–102, 1988.

D35 Warren, J.A. *et al.*: PAA film application and the amalgam-PAA-glass ionomer bond, Dent. Mater. 4: 338–340, 1988.

D36 Barakat, M.M. *et al.*: Parameters that affect *in vitro* bonding of glass-ionomer liners to dentin, J. Dent. Res. 67(9): 1161–1163, 1988.

D37 Maniatopoulos, C. *et al.*: Evaluation of shear strength at the cement-endodontic post interface, J. Prosthet. Dent. 59(6): 662–668, 1988.

D38 Kakaboura, A. *et al.*: The effect of an air-powder abrasive device on the bond strength of glass ionomer cements to dentin, Quintessence Int. 20(1): 9–12, 1989.

D39 Hinoura, K. *et al.*: Effect of the bonding agent on the bond strength between glass ionomer cement and composite resin, Quintessence Int. 20(1): 31–35, 1989.

E.   Solubility·Water Sensitivity

E1   Crisp, S. *et al.*: Glass ionomer cements, chemistry of erosion, J. Dent. Res. 55: 1032–1041, 1976.

E2   Hirabayashi, S.: Composition and solubility of glass-ionomer cement, J. Dent. 3: 24–25, 1987. (Japanese)

E3   Saito, S.: Characteristic and clinical of glass-ionomer cement, Part 1 Study on relation to hardening process and water. J. Dent. Med. 8(4): 456–468, 1978. (Japanese)

E4   Mitchem, J.C., and Gronas, D.G.: Clinical evaluation of cement solubility, J. prosthet. Dent. 40(4): 453–456, 1978.

E5   Saito, S.: Passage a progress report of glass-ionomer cement, J. Dent. Med. 10(1): 104–125, 1979. (Japanese)

E6   Okamoto, S. *et al.*: Surface crack of glass-ionomer cement. Part 1 Change of humidity and temperature J.J. Conserv. Dent. 22(1): 195–196, 1979. (Japanese)

E7   Kota, K. *et al.*: Chalky appearance with surface erosion of the glass-ionomer cement, J.J. Conserv. Dent. 23(2): 584–590, 1980. (Japanese)

E8   Saito, S.: Clinical part of glass-ionomer cement, J.J. Conserv. Dent. 24(3): 1105–1106, 1981. (Japanese)

E9   Okamoto, S. *et al.*: Surface crack of glass-ionomer cement, J.J. Conserv. Dent. 35(1): 123–128, 1981. (Japanese)

E10   Mitchem, J.C., and Gronas, D.G.: Continued evaluation of the clinical solubility of luting cements, J. Prosthet. Dent. 45(3): 289–291, 1981.

E11   Mesu, F.P.: Degradation of luting cements measured *in vitro*, J. Dent. Res. 61(5): 665–672, 1982.

E12   Beech, D.R., and Bandyopadhyay, S.: A new laboratory method for evaluating the relative solubility and erosion of dental cements, J. Oral Rehabil. 10: 57–63, 1983.

E13   Sidler, P., and Strub, J.R.: *In-vivo*-untersuchung der löslichkeit und des abdichtungsvermögens von drei befestigungzementen, Dtsch. Zahnarztl. Z. 38: 564–571, 1983.

E14   Matsuie, S. *et al.*: Passage a progress resort of glass-ionomer cement for organic acid erosion, J. Dent. Mater. 3(2): 210–219, 1984. (Japanese)

E15   Jean-Francois Roulet, and Christian Walti: Influence of oral fluids composite resin and glass-ionomer cement, J. Prosthet. Dent. 52(2): 182–189, 1984.

E16   Omori, H. *et al.*: Experiment of water sensitivity to glass ionomer cement, J. Michinoku Dent. Soci. 16: 1–2, 92–95, 1985. (Japanese)

E17   Setchell, D.J. *et al.*: The relative solubilities of four modern glass-ionomer cements, Br. Dent. J. 158(6): 220–222, 1985.

E18   A Sensitive conductimetric method for measuring the material initially water leache from dental cements, J. Dent. 14: 74–79, 1986.

E19 Earl, M.S.A., and Ibbetson, R.J.: The clinical disintegration of a glass-ionomer cement, Br. Dent. J. 161(8): 287–291, 1986.

E20 Saito, S. *et al.*: Study on water sensitivity for glass-ionomer cement, J.J. Conserv. Dent. 30: 92, 1987. (Japanese)

E21 Pluim, L.J., and Arends, J.: The relation between salivary properties and *in vivo* solubility of dental cements, Dent. Mater. 3: 13–18, 1987.

E22 Phillips, R.W. *et al.*: *In vivo* disintegration of luting cements, J.A.D.A. Apr. 114: 489–492, 1987.

E23 Ando, M.: Elution of lutin cement for organic acid J.J. Prosth. Soc. 32(1): 203–217, 1988. (Japanese)

E24 Tsuchio, H., and Yoshida, T.: Disintegration and solution experiment of dental materials—Elusion of structure materials for luting cement, J.J. Dent. Ass. 41(6): 619–631, 1988. (Japanese)

E25 Walls, A.W.G. *et al.*: The effect of the variation in pH of the eroding solution upon the erosion resistance of glass polyalkenoate (ionomer) cement, Br. Dent. J. 5: 141–144, 1988.

F.   Biological Affinity

F1   Phillips, R.W., and Swartz, M.L.: Effect of certain restorative materials on solubility of enamel, J.A.D.A. 54: 623–636, 1957.

F2   Mericle, M.R., and Muhler, J.C.: Studies concerning the antisolubility effectiveness of different stannous fluoride prophylaxis paste mixtures, J. Dent. Res. 42: 21–27, 1963.

F3   Lind, V. *et al.*: Contact caries in connection with silver amalgam, copper amalgam and silicate fillings, Acta. Odontl. Scand. 22: 333–341, 1964.

F4   Phillips, R.W.: Materials for the practicing dentist, 1969, C.V. Mosby Co.

F5   Ingram, B.L.: Determination of fluoride in silicate rocks without separation of aluminum using a specific ion electrode, Anal. Chem. 42: 1825–1827, 1970.

F6   Forsten, L., and Paunio, I.K.: Fluoride release by silicate cements and composite resins, Scand. J. Dent. Res. 80: 515–519, 1972.

F7   Norman, R.D. *et al.*: Effects of restorative materials on plaque composition, J. Dent. Res. 51: 1596–1601, 1972.

F8   Munksgaard, E.C., and Bruun, C.: Determination of fluoride in superficial enamel biopsies from human teeth by means of gas chromatography, Archs. Oral. Biol. 18: 735–744, 1973.

F9   Forsten, L., and Paunio, I.K.: Fluoride release from varnish-coated silicates and from cavity liners and fissure sealants, Scand. J. Dent. Res. 81: 513–517, 1973.

F10 Crips, S., and Wilson, A.D.: Reactions in glass ionomer cements. I. Decomposition of the powder, J. Dent. Res. 53: 1408–1413, 1974.

F11 Crips, S., and Wilson, A.D.: Reactions in glass ionomer cements. III. The Precipitation reaction, J. Dent. Res. 53: 1420–1424, 1974.

F12 Klotzer, W.T.: Pulp reaction to a glass ionomer cement, J. Dent. Res. 54: 678, 1975.

F13 Dahl, B.L., and Tronstad, L.: Biological tests of an experimental glass ionomer cement, J. Oral. Rehabil. 3: 19, 1976.

F14 Imanishi, Y. *et al.*: Study on cytotoxy of glass-ionomer cements (*In vitro*) J.J. Dent. App. mater. 5: 40–41, 1977. (Japanese)

F15 Onose, H. *et al.*: Study on the antibacterial effects of the glass-ionomer cement, J.J. Conserv. Dent. 20(2): 406–409, 1977. (Japanese)

F16 Koulourides, T., and Axelsson, P.: Experiment and clinical studies of caries arrestment, Caries Res. 11: 130, 1977.

F17 Forsten, L.: Fluoride release from a glass ionomer cement, Scand. J. Dent. Res. 85: 503–504, 1977.

F18 Onose, H. *et al.*: Study on the antibacterial effects of the glass ionomer cement, Biocompatibility Dent. Mater. 20: 130, 1977. (Japanese)

F19 Yakushiji, H. *et al.*: Effects of glass-ionomer cement on human dental pulp and its pulp protection under composite resin restoration, J. Pedodont. 16(3): 521–528, 1978. (Japanese)

F20 Yoshiiri, K. *et al.*: Influence of cement's electric resistance and change of elution pH for pulp, J. Dent. Med. 8(4): 469–478, 1978. (Japanese)

F21 Tobias, R.S. *et al.*: Pulpal response to a glass ionomer cement, Br. Dent. J. 144: 345–350, 1978.

F22 Sogawa, K.: Investigate the cause for glass-ionomer cement's cytotoxy, Dentist. 42(6): 761–762, 1979. (Japanese)

F23 Kimura, M. *et al.*: Experiment of glass-ionomer cement for pulp tissue changes, J. Dent. Med. 9(1): 88–94, 1979. (Japanese)

F24 Yakushiji, H. *et al.*: Influence of glass-ionomer cement for pulp and indirect pulp capping, J. Tokyo Dent. Coll. Soci. 79(3): 641–642, 1979. (Japanese)

F25 Saito, S.: The pulp damage actions, Dent. diamond 4(10): 69–72, 1979. (Japanese)

F26 Nakagaki, H.: Basic studies on human enamel biopsy. Part 1. Measurement of enamel solubility, J. Dent. Heal. 28: 26–59, 1979. (Japanese)

F27 Kawahara, H. *et al.*: Judge of tissue stimulus by culture tissue material, Dent. diamond 4(11): 67–70, 1979. (Japanese)

F28 Hotz, P.R.: Experimental secondary caries around amalgam composite and glass ionomer cement fillings in Human teeth, Helvetica Odontological Acta. Sep. 23: 9–39, 1979.

F29 Putt, M.S. *et al.*: Studies of prophylaxis pastes containing sodium-potassium aluminum silicate and fluoride, J. Dent. Res. 58: 1659–1663, 1979.

F30 Council on dental materials and devices (Association Reports). Status report on the glass ionomer cements, J.A.D.A. 99: 221–226, 1979.

F31 Kawahara, H. *et al.*: Biological evaluation on glass-ionomer cements, J. Dent. Res. 58: 1080–1086, 1979.

F32 Ishikawa, T.: Pulp reaction of new esthetic restorative materials, Dent. Revi. Oct. 456: 71–76, 1980. (Japanese)

F33 Ohashi, T. *et al.*: Influence of fuji ionomer (Type I) for pathological findings of dental pulps, J. Tokyo Dent. Coll. Soci. 80(6): 929–939, 1980. (Japanese)

F34 Koulourides, T. *et al.*: Enhancement of fluoride effectiveness by experimental cariogenic priming of human enamel, Caries Res. 14: 32–39, 1980.

F35 Feagin, F. *et al.*: Effects of fluoride in remineralized human surface enamel on dissolution resistance, J. Dent. Res. 59: 1016–1071, 1980.

F36 Swartz, J.L. *et al.*: Fluoride distribution in teeth using a silicate model, J. Dent. Res. 59(10): 1596–1603, 1980.

F37 Mellbeng, J.R.: Rate of fluoride uptake by surface and subsurface sound enamel from monofluorophosphate, Caries Res. 14: 50–55, 1980.

F38 Wesenberg, G., and Hals, E.: The *in vitro* effect of a glass ionomer cement on dentine and enamel walls, J. Oral. Rehabil. 7: 35–42, 1980.

F39 Wesenberg, G., and Hals, E.: The structure of experimental *in vitro* lesions around glass ionomer cement restoration in human teeth, J. Oral. Rehabil. 7: 175–184, 1980.

F40 Sogawa, K.: Comparative study on cytotoxy of main components of three luting cements (*in vitro*), J.J. Dent. App. Mater. 22(59): 172–186, 1981. (Japanese)

F41 Komatsu, H.: Glass-ionomer cement for caries prevention. Effect of fluoride content on acid resistance of human enamel, J. Conserv. Dent. 24(3): 814–826, 1981. (Japanese)

F42 Ohasi, T. *et al.*: Pathologic experimental of effect to pulp by fuji Ionomer type 1. J.J. Conserv. Dent. 24(3): 1105, 1981. (Japanese)

F43 Ishikawa, I., and Noro, A.: Pulp rectio some kind of dental restorative materials. J.J. Dent. Ass. 34(9): 914–924, 1981. (Japanese)

F44 Hanks, C.T. *et al.*: Cytotoxic effects of dental cements on two cell culture systems, J. Oral Pathology. 10: 101–112, 1981.

F45 Bjorgtveit, A., and Gjerdet, N.R.: Fluoride release from a fluoride-containing amalgam, a glass ionomer cement and a silicate cement in artificial saliva, J. Oral. Rehabil. 8: 237–241, 1981.

F46 Paterson, R.C., and Watts, A.: The response of the rat molar pulp to a glass ionomer cement, Br. Dent. J. 151(7): 228–230, 1981.

F47 Pameijer, C.H. *et al.*: Pulpal response to a glass-ionomer cement in primates, J. Prosthet. Dent. 46(1): 36–40, 1981.

F48 Nakamura, M. *et al.*: Father studies on long-term biocomputibility test of composite resins and Ionomer Cement. J.J. Conserv. Dent. 25(3): 667–680, 1982. (Japanese)

F49 Hotta, D. *et al.*: Influence of the glass-ionomer cement on deciduous Pulp. J.J. Pedodont. 16(3): 521–528, 1978. (Japanese)

F50 Komatsu, H.: Change of acid proof of enamel for glass-ionomer cement, J. Dent. Med. 15(5): 626–627, 1982. (Japanese)

F51 Sato, N. *et al.*: The antibacterial activity of dental restorative materials, J.J. Conserv. Dent. 25(2): 442–452, 1982. (Japanese)

F52 Cranfield, M. *et al.*: Factors relating to the rate of fluoride-ion release from glass ionomer cement, J. Dent. 10(4): 333–341, 1982.

F53 Derkson, G.D. *et al.*: Fluoride release from a silicophosphate cement with added fluoride, J. Dent. Res. 61(5): 660–664, 1982.

F54 Imai, Y. *et al.*: Evaluation of the biologic effects of dental materials using a new cell culture technique, J. Dent. Res. 61(8): 1024–1027, 1982.

F55 Bartels, T. *et al.*: Fluoridation of human enamel by fluoride containing polyelectrolytes, Caries Res. 16: 57–63, 1982.

F56 Chander, S. *et al.*: Transformation of calcium fluoride for caries prevention, J. Dent. Res. 61: 403–407, 1982.

F57 Tanase, S.: Effect of glass-ionomer cement on occurrence of Recurrent Caries, J. Pedodont. 21(3) 426–440, 1983. (Japanese)

F58 Tsujimura, I.: Influence of pulp for Combined for tannin and fluorine for cements, J. Tokyo Dent. Coll. Soci. 83: 891–935, 1983. (Japanese)

F59 Meryon, S.D. *et al.*: A comparison of the *in vitro* cytotoxicity of two glass-ionomer cements, J. Dent. Res. 62(6): 769–773, 1983.

F60 Dijkman, A.G. *et al. In vivo* investigation on the fluoride content in and on human enamel after typical applications, Caries Res. 17: 392–402, 1983.

F61 Bruun, C. *et al.*: Study on the dissolution behaviour of calcium fluoride, Scand. J. Dent. Res. 91: 247–250, 1983.

F62 Zmener, O., and Dominguez, F.V.: Tissure response to a glass ionomer used as an endodontic cement, A preliminary study in dogs, Oral Surg. 56(2): 198–205, 1983.

F63 Yoshida, S.: Inhibitory action of glass-ionomer cement for recurrent caries, Dent. Diamond 9(5): 42–43, 1984. (Japanese)

F64 Ota, Y. *et al.*: Antibacterial effect of plastic filling materials. J. Tokyo Dent. Coll. Soci. 84(1): 83–88, 1984. (Japanese)

F65 Meryon, S.D., and Smith, A.J.: A comparison of fluoride release from three glass ionomer cements and a polycarboxylate cement, Int. Endod. J. 17: 16–24, 1984.

F66 Rosen, S. *et al.*: Anticariogenic effects of tea in rats, J. Dent. Res. 63: 658–660, 1984.

F67 Retief, D.H. *et al.*: Enamel and cementum fluoride uptake from a glass ionomer cement, Caries Res. 18: 250–257, 1984.

F68 Derand, T., and Johansson, B.: Experimental secondary caries around restorations in roots, Caries Res. 18: 548–554, 1984.

F69 Staehle, H.J., and Bobmann, K.: Experimentelle untersuchungen über die antikariognne wirkung von glasionomerzement, Dtsch. Zahnärztl. Z. 39(7): 532–534, 1984.

F70 Swartz, M.L. *et al.*: Long-term f release from glass ionomer cements, J. Dent. Res. 63(2): 158–160, 1984.

F71 Plant, C.G. *et al.*: Pulpal effects of glass ionomer cements, Int. Endod. J. 17: 51–59, 1984.

F72 Reported sensitivity to glass ionomer luting cements, J.A.D.A. 109(Sep): 476, 1984.

F73 Maebara, S.: Cytotoxicity composite resin and glass-ionomer cement for HELA S-3 cell, J. Biomed. Mater. Res. 3(1): 27–43, 1985. (Japanese)

F74 Kawada, Y.: Influence of dental cements for HELA S-3 cell, J. Biomed. Mater. Res. 3(4): 49–61, 1985. (Japanese)

F75 Saitoh, S.: Protect the pulp, Quintessence 4: 5–11, 1985. (Japanese)

F76 Kimura, M. *et al.*: Pathological exploration of stimulation to pulp for lining cement, J. Dent. Med. 22(3): 329–336, 1985. (Japanese)

F77 Skartveit, L. *et al.*: Fluoride release from a fluoride containing amalgam *in vivo*, Scand. J. Dent. Res. 93: 448–452, 1985.

F78 Tung, M.s. *et al.*: Hydrolysis of dicalcium phosphate dihydrate in the presence or absence of calcium fluoride, J. Dent. Res. 64: 2–5, 1985.

F79 Ohashi, T.: Pulpal response of human dentalpulp to glass-ionomer cements. (Fuji ionomer Type I & II), J.J. Conserv. Dent, 29(2): 33–68, 1986. (Japanese)

F80 Yasuda, A.: The influence of decomposition and saliva's pH for glass-ionomer cement, J. Tokyo Dent. Coll. Soci. 74(4) 858–873, 1986. (Japanese)

F81 Smith, D.C., and Ruse, N.D.: Acidity of glass ionomer cements during setting and its relation to pulp sensitivity, J.A.D.A. 122: 654–657, 1986.

F82 Schmalz, G. *et al.*: Die pulpavertraglichkeit eines glasionomer-und eines zinkoxiphos phat-zementes, Dtsch. Zahnärztl. Z. 41(8): 806–812, 1986.

F83 Klotzer, W.T., and Schmalz, G.: Din-Vornorm 13930: Biologische prüfung von dentalwerkstoffen, Dtsch. Zahanarztl Z. 41(12): 1248–1252, 1986.

F84 Thornton, J.B., *et al.*: Fluoride release from and tensile bond strength of Ketac-Fil and Ketac-Silver to enamel and dentin, Dent. Mater. 2: 241–245, 1986.

F85 Thylstrup, A., and Fejerskov, O.: Textbook of cariology, Munksgaard, Copenhagen, 38, 1986.

188

F86 Thylstrup, A., and Fejerskov, O.: Textbook of cariology, Munksgaard, Copenhagen, 183, 1986.

F87 Thylstrup, A., and Fejerskov, O.: Textbook of cariology, Munksgaard, Copenhagen, 193–194, 1986.

F88 Prosser, H.J., *et al.*: Glass-ionomer cements of improved flexural strength, J. Dent. Res. 65: 146–148, 1986.

F89 Yamamoto, K. *et al.*: Antibiotic effects of dental cements on oral bacteria, J.J. Conserv. Dent, 30(6): 1551–1555, 1987. (Japanese)

F90 Ishikawa, T.: Adhesive resin and pulp protection, Dent. Rev. Aug. 538: 79–90, 1987. (Japanese)

F91 Okamoto, A. *et al.*: The influence of glass ionomer cements used for base of lining to dentin, Part 1. pH changes in glass-ionomer cements, J.J. Conserv. Dent. 30(5): 1401–1406, 1987. (Japanese)

F92 Heys, R.J. *et al.*: An evaluation of a glass ionomer lutingagent: pulpal histological response, J.A.D.A. 114, 607–611, 1987.

F93 Schmalz, G.: Antimikrobielle eigenschaften eines zinkoxiphosphat-zementes und eines glasionomer-zementes mit und ohne slberzusatz, Dtsch. Zahnarztl. Z. 42(7): 628–632, 1987.

F94 McCombe, D., and Ericson, D.: Antimicrobial action of new, proprietary lining cements, J. Dent. Res. 66(5): 1025–1028, 1987.

F95 Fitzgerald, M. *et al.*: An evaluation of a glass ionomer luting agent. Bacterial Leakage, J.A.D.A. 114(June): 783–786, 1987.

F96 Hattab, F.N.: Direct determination of fluoride in selected dental materials, Dent. Mater. 3(2): 67–70, 1987.

F97 Fukazawa, M. *et al.*: Mechanism for erosion of glass-ionomer cements in an acidic buffer solution, J. Dent. Res. 66: 1770–1774, 1987.

F98 Paterson, R.C., and Watts, A.: Toxicity to the pulp of a glass-ionomer cement, Br. Dent. J. 163(3): 110–112, 1987.

F99 Meryon, S.D., and Jakeman, K.J.: Uptake of zinc and fluoride by several dentin components, J. Biomed. Mater. Res. 21(1): 127–135, 1987.

F100 Willershausen, B. *et al.*: Versuche mit glasionomerzenmenten in der zellkultur bel längerer liegezeit, Dtsch. Zahnarztl. Z. 42(4): 342–344, 1987.

F101 Tominaga, N. *et al.*: Antibacterial effect and cytotoxicity of certain pulp capping materials, J.J. Conserv. Dent. 31(4): 1194–1201, 1988. (Japanese)

F102 Fujii, B.: Relativity of lining materials for pulp, J. Tokyo Dent. Ass. 6(4): 251–255, 1988. (Japanese)

F103 Yamamoto, K. *et al.*: Antibacterial effects of temporary cements on oral bacteria, J.J. Conserv. Dent. 31(4): 1114–1117, 1988. (Japanese)

F104 Strubig, W.: Fluoridaufnahme im zahnzchmeiz aus glasionomerzementen, Dtsch. Zahnarztl. Z. 43(7): 789–791, 1988.

F105 Muzynski, B.L. *et al.*: Fluoride release from glass ionomer used as luting agents, J. Prosthet. Dent. 60(1): 41–44, 1988.

F106 Restorative materials containing fluoride, J.A.D.A. (Association Report). 116(6): 762–763, 1988.

F107 Oshima, K. *et al.*: The change of fluoride concentration in enamel after removal glassionomer cement by *in vivo*, J.J. Conserv. Dent. 32: 986–993, 1989. (Japanese)

F108 Fujibayashi, S. *et al.*: Fluorine's content and elution of dental cement J. Hokkaido Dent. Ass. 44: 277–285, 1989. (Japanese)

G. Marginal Sealing

G1 Ohkawa, A.: Studies on marginal closure of various restorative materials, especially, on the leakage properties related to the cavity outline form. J.J. Conserv. Dent. 22(2): 225–248, 1979. (Japanese)

G2 Shimokobe, H. *et al.*: Study on marginal adaptation of glass-ionomer cement fillings, J.J. Conserv. Dent. 21:(1): 94–101, 1978. (Japanese)

G3 Kidd, E.A.M.: Cavity sealing ability of composite and glass-ionomer cement restorations: An assessment *in vitro*, Br. Dent. J. 144(5): 139–142, 1978.

G4 Hembree, J.H., and Andrews, J.T.: Microleakage of several class V anterior restorative materials, A laboratory study, J.A.D.A. 97: 179–183, 1978.

G5 Fuks, A.B. *et al.*: Marginal adaptation of glassionomer cements, J. Prosthet. Dent. 49(3): 356–360, 1983.

G6 Myers, M.L. *et al.*: Marginal leakage of contemporary cementing agents, J. Prosthet. Dent. 50(4): 513–515, 1983.

G7 Alperstein, K.S. *et al.*: Marginal leakage of glass ionomer cement restorations, J. Prosthet. Dent. 50: 803–807, 1983.

G8 Brandau, H.E. *et al*.: Restoration of cervical contours on nonprepared teeth using glass ionomer cements; a 4½ year report, J.A.D.A. 104: 782–783, 1984.

G9 Mount, G.J.: Readers' round table, J. Prosthet. Dent. 51(6): 854, 1984.

G10 Gordon, M. *et al*.: Microleakage of four composite resins over a glass ionomer cement base in class V restorations, Quintessence Int. 12: 817–820, 1985.

G11 Welsh E.L., and Hembree, J.H.: Micro-leakage at the gingival wall with four class V anterior restorative materials, J. Prosthet. Dent. 54: 370–372, 1985.

G12 Van Dijken, J.W.V., and Horstedt, P.: *In vivo* adaptation of restorative materials to dentin, J. Prosthet. Dent. 56(6): 677–681, 1986.

G13 Assessment of microleakage of restorative materials by a diffusion model, J. Oral. Rehabil. 13: 355–363, 1986.

G14 Tyas, M.J.: Clinical evaluation of Scotchbond, one year results, Aust. Dent. J. 31: 159–164, 1986.

G15 Irie, M.: Relativity of marginal shut and physical properties for dental restorative glass-ionomer cement, J.J. Conserv. Dent. 30(2): 764–765, 1987. (Japanese)

G16 Ziemieckl, T.L. *et al*.: Clinical evaluation of cervical composite resin restorations placed without retention, Oper. Dent. 12: 27–33, 1987.

G17 Shimizu, A. *et al*.: Microleakage of amalgam restoration with adhesive resin cement, Dent. Mater. 6(1): 64–69, 1987.

G18 Van Dijken, J.W.V., and Horstedt, P.: Effects of 5% sodium hypochlorite or tubulicid pre-treatment *in vivo* on the marginal adaptation of dental adhesives and glass ionomer cements, Dent. Mater. 3(6): 303–306, 1987.

G19 Hotta, M.: Marginal sealing of visible light-cured composite resins in cervical cavities, J.J. Conserv. Dent. 31(5): 1371–1388, 1988. (Japanese)

G20 Robbins, J.W., and Cooley, R.L.: Microleakage of Ketac-Silver in the tunnel preparation, Oper. Dent. 13: 8–11, 1988.

G21 Wenner, K.K. *et al*.: Microleakage of root restorations, J.A.D.A. 117(7): 825–828, 1988.

G22 Haller, B. *et al*.: Der einflu β von kavitätenrandbearbeitung und kavitätenreinigung auf die dichtheit zervikaler glasionomerzement-füllongen, Dtsch. Zahnarztl. Z. 43(8): 933–938, 1988.

G23 Shortall, A.C. *et al*.: Marginal seal of injection-molded ceramic crowns cemented with three adhesive systems, J. Prosthet. Dent. 61(1): 24–27, 1989.

G24 Hembree, J.H.: Microleakage at the gingival margin of class II composite restorations with glass-ionomer liner, J. Prosthet. Dent. 61(1): 28–30, 1989.

H. Clinical Use and Criterion

H1 Saito, S.: Valuation of glass-ionomer cement, Int. J. Dent. Med. 6(2): 167–185, 1977. (Japanese)

H2 Hashimoto, K. *et al*.: Cautions for handling of glass-ionomer cement, Dent. Rev. Dec, 422: 79–89, 1977. (Japanese)

H3 Plant, C.G. *et al*.: The use of a glass ionomer cement in deciduous teeth, Br. Dent. J. 143(8): 271–274, 1977.

H4 Saito, S.: Clinical studies on glass-ionomer cement, Int. J. Dent. Med. 6: 167, 1977. (Japanese)

H5 Hashimoto, K., and Irie, M.: How to use and problem of glass-ionomer cement, Dent. Rev. 430: 37–42, 1978. (Japanese)

H6 Mount, G.J., and Makinson, O.: Clinical characteristics of a glass-ionomer cement, Br. Dent. J. 145(3): 67–71, 1978.

H7 Saito, S.: Indicate and clinical care of glass-ionomer cements, Dent. Outlook 54(5): 793–807, 1979. (Japanese)

H8 Tomitani, J.: Studies on the finishing or polishing procedures of glass-ionomer cement restoration, J.J. Conserv. Dent. 23(2): 255–289, 1980. (Japanese)

H9 Shimizu, T. *et al*.: Influence of lubricants on finishing and polishing surface roughness of glass-ionomer cement, J.J. Conserv. Dent. 23(2): 347–350, 1980. (Japanese)

H10 Saito, S.: Clinic and character of glass-ionomer cement effect of reduction in initial harding time, J. Dent. Med. 12(6): 725–735, 1980. (Japanese)

H11 Saito, S.: Clinic and character of glass-ionomer cement, Dent. Diamond 5(1): 69–72, 1980. (Japanese)

H12 Yakusiji, H.: The application of glass-ionomer cement to pedodontics, Dent. Outlook 56(5): 687–698, 1980. (Japanese)

H13 Saito, S. *et al*.: Revaluation of glass-ionomer cement —plastic materials—, Dent. Outlook 57(1): 145–162, 1981. (Japanese)

H14 Smales, R.J.: Clinical use of ASPA glass-ionomer cement, Br. Dent. J. 151(2): 58–60, 1981.

H15 Seluk, L.W., and Smith, F.W.: Use of a glass ionomer cement restorative, J. Michigan Dent. Assoc. 63: 265–267, 1981.

H16 Reisbick, M.H.: Working qualities of glass-ionomer cements, J. Prosthet. Dent. 46(5): 525–529, 1981.

H17 Lampert, V.F.: Glasionomerzement als Füllungsmaterial für den zahnhals, Dtsch. Zahnarztl. Z. 37(2): 191–193, 1982.

H18 Results of CRA consumer opinion survey, C.R.A. Newsletter. 6: issue. 3-Mar. 1982.

H19 Katsuyama, S.: Cavity of glass-ionomer cement. Improvement of adhesive property and cavity form, Dent. Outlook 91–98, 1983. (Japanese)

H20 Kawami, T. et al.: Operative dentistry. The application of the glass-ionomer cement to clinic, Dent. Diamond 8(12): 38–39, 1983. (Japanese)

H21 Saito, S.: Operative dentistry of milk teeth. Consideration of adhesive material for clinical progress, Dent. Outlook 2: 273–280, 1983. (Japanese)

H22 Glass ionomer restorative materials, C.R.A. Newsletter. 7: issue. 6-Jun. 1983.

H23 Pearson, G.J.: Finishing of glass-ionomer cements, Br. Dent. J. 155: 226–228, 1983.

H24 Katsuyama, S. et al.: Clinical technique and care of glass-ionomer cement, Dent. Diamond 9(14): 56–61, 1984. (Japanese)

H25 Fuks, A.B. et al.: Clinical evaluation of a glass-ionomer cement used as a class II restorative material in primary molars, J. Pedodont. 8: 393–399, 1984.

H26 Knibbs, P.J., and Pearson, G.J.: Finishing glass-ionomer cement, Br. Dent. J. 157(11): 398–400, 1984.

H27 Mount, G.J.: Glass ionomer cements, clinical considerations, Clinical Dentistry 20A(D-8): 1–23, 1984.

H28 Hunt, P.R.: A modified class II cavity preparation for glass ionomer restorative materials, Quintessence Int. 10: 1011–1018, 1984.

H29 Saito, S.: Study on clinical time—related for glass-ionomer cement, J.J. Conserv. Dent. 29(3): 1066, 1986. (Japanese)

H30 Knibbs, P.J., and Plant, C.G.: A clinical assessment of a rapid setting glass-ionomer cement, Br. Dent. J. 161(9): 323–326, 1986.

H31 A clinical assessment of an anhydrous glass ionomer cement, Br. Dent. J. (Aug): 99–103, 1986.

H32 Staehle, H.J.: Experimentelle und klinische studie über verschiedene glasionomerzemente, Dtsch. Zahnarztl. Z. 41(2): 195–199, 1986.

H33 Monteiro, S. et al.: Evaluation of materials and techniques for restoration of erosion areas, J. Prosthet. Dent. 55(4): 434, 1986.

H34 Ngo, H. et al.: Glass-ionomer cements, A 12-month evaluation, J. Prosthet. Dent. 55(2): 203–205, 1986.

H35 Foreman, F.J., and Theobald, W.D.: Direct bonded glass ionomer crowns, J. Dent. Child. 54(3): 165–169, 1987.

H36 Technical report No.27: Guide to the use of glass ionomer filling materials federation dentaire internationale, Int. Dent. J. 37(3): 183–184, 1987.

H37 Berry, E.A., and Berry L.L.: The successful use of glass ionomer luting cements without post-cementation sensitivity, Texas Dent. J. (Feb): 8–11, 1987.

H38 Hickel, R., and Vob, A.: Untersuchungen zur tunnelpräparation, Dtsch. Zahnarztl. Z. 42(6): 545–548, 1987.

H39 Walls, A.W.G. et al.: The use of glass polyalkenoate(ionomer) cements in the deciduous dentition, Br. Dent. J. 165(1): 13–17, 1988.

H40 Hill, F.J., and Halaseh, F.J.: A laboratory investigation of tunnel restorations in premolar teeth, Br. Dent. J. 165(10): 364–367, 1988.

H41 Matis, B.A. et al.: Clinical evaluation and early finishing of glass ionomer restorative materials, Oper. Dent. 13: 74–80, 1988.

H42 Woolford, M.J.: Finishing glass polyalkenoate (glass-ionomer) cements, Br. Dent. J. 165(11): 395–399, 1988.

H43 Mizrahi, E.: Glass ionomer cements in orthodontics—an update, American J. Orthod. Dentofac. Orthop. 93(6): 505–507, 1988.

H44 Engelsmann, U. et al.: Vergleichende langzeituntersuchung über die füllungsmaterialien Ketac Fil und amalgam an milchzähnen, Dtsch. Zahnarztl. Z. 43(3): 291–294, 1988.

I. Application for Cementation

I1 Wilson, A.D. et al.: Experimental luting agents based on the glass-ionomer cements, Br. Dent. J. 142: 117–122, 1977.

I2 Kimura, K. et al.: Rise of cast crown for glass-ionomer cement 25(2): 304–310, 1981. (Japanese)

I3 Reisbick, M.H.: Working qualities of glass ionomer cements, J. Prosthet. Dent. 46(5): 525–530, 1981.

I4 McCamb, D.: Retention of castings with glass ionomer cements, J. Prosthet. Dent. 48(3): 285–291, 1982.

I5 Endo, T.: A study on the dental cement for luting, 2. Retention force and some other characteristics of luting cements, J.J. Conserv. Dent. 26(1): 11–27, 1983. (Japanese)

I6 McLean, W. et al.: Development and use of water-hardening glass-ionomer luting cements, J. Prosthet. Dent. 52: 175–181, 1984.

I7 Brose, N.O. et al.: Internal channel vents for posterior complete crowns, J. Prosthet. Dent. 51(6): 755–760, 1984.

I8 Fricker, J.P., and McLachian, M.D.: Clinical studies of glass ionomer cements part 1. glass ionomer zinc, Aust. Orthod. J. Mar(9): 179–180, 1985.

I9 Fricker, J.P., and McLachian, M.D.: Clinical studies of glass ionomer cements part 2. Aust. Orthod. J. Mar(10): 12–14, 1987.

I10 Foreman, F.J., and Theobald, W.D.: Direct bonded glass ionomer crowns, J. Dent. Child. 54(3): 165–169, 1987.

I11 Tjan, A.H.L. et al.: Effects of various cementation methods on the retention of prefabricated posts, J. Prosthet. Dent. 58(3): 309–313, 1987.

I12 Kobayashi, K. et al.: Luting cement, Dent. Outlook 72(6): 1281–1286, 1988. (Japanese)

I13 Rosenstiel, S.F., and Gegauff, A.G.: Improving the cementation of complete cast crowns: A comparison of static and dynamic seating methods, J.A.D.A. 117: 845–848, 1988.

I14 Plant, C.G. et al.: Pulpal response to a glass-ionomer luting cement, Br. Dent. J. 165(2): 54–58, 1988.

J. Application for Class III, Class V and Root Surface Filling

J1 Lawrence, L.G.: Cervical glass ionomer restorations. A clinical study, J. Can. Dent. Assoc. 45: 58, 1979.

J2 Ishikawa, T.: Treatment of cervical caries for old man use of glass-ionomer cement, Dent. Outlook 60(2): 257–267, 1982. (Japanese)

J3 Saito, S.: Treatment and adhesion of root surface caries with age, Dent. Outlook 2: 130–137, 1983. (Japanese)

J4 Goto, T. et al.: Countermeasure of old man's rootsurface caries, Dent. Rev. 489: 113–122, 1983. (Japanese)

J5 Shimizu, A. et al.: Clinical experiment of treatment method for hypersensitivity, J. Osaka Univ. Dent. Soc. 29(2): 362–367, 1984. (Japanese)

J6 Brandau, H.E. et al.: Restoration of cervical contours on nonprepared teeth using glass-ionomer cement, A four and one half-year, J.A.D.A. 104(May): 782–783, 1984.

J7 Kullmann, W.: Dentinhaft-komposit und glasionomer-zemente zur restauration zervikaler läsionen, Dtsch. Zahnarztl. Z. 40: 922–926, 1985.

J8 Osborne, J.W., and Berry, T.G.: Clinical assessment of glass ionomer cements as class III restorations. A one-year report, Dent. Mater. 2: 147–150, 1986.

J9 Norman, C.: Bitter glass ionomer-microfil technique for restoring cervical lesions, J. Prosthet. Dent. 55(6): 661–662, 1986.

J10 Onose, H. et al.: Dental esthetic restoration of discolored tooth. Root surface carries of old man, Dent. Enginee. 83: 10–13, 1987. (Japanese)

J11 Knibbs, P.J.: A clinical report on the use of a glass ionomer cement to restore cervical margin lesions, J. Oral. Rehabil. 14: 105–109, 1987.

J12 Haller, B. et al.: Der einfluss von glasionomer-zementen und dentinadhaesiven auf die randständigkeit zervikaler kompositfüllungen, Dtsch. Zahnarztl. Z. 42(6): 588–593, 1987.

J13 Voss, A., and Hickel, R.: Nachuntersuchung von zervikaren glasionomerzemente und kompositfüllungen, Dtsch. Zahnarztl. Z. 43(8): 944–946, 1988.

K. Lining and Base

K1 McLean, J.W., and Wilson, A.D.: The clinical development of the glass ionomer cements. Aust. Dent. J. 22(2): 120–127, 1977.

K2 Murray, G.A., and Yates, J.L.: A comparison of the bond strengths of composite resins and glass ionomer cement, J. Pedodont. 8: 172–177, 1984.

K3 Influence of oral fluid on composite resin and glass-ionomer cement, J. Prosthet. Dent. Aug. 52(2): 182–189, 1984.

K4 McLean, J.W. et al.: The use of glass-ionomer cements in bonding composite resins to dentine, Br. Dent. J. 158(11): 410–414, 1985.

K5 Sneed, W.D., and Looper, S.W.: Shere bond strength of a composite resin to an etched glass ionomer, Dent. Mater. 1: 127–128, 1985.

K6 Base or liner, C.R.A. Newsletter. 9: issue. 3-Mar. 1985.

K7 Tunoda, M.: Influence and pulp protection light cure composite resin restoration, J. Tokyo Dent. Coll. Soci. 627–673, 1986. (Japanese)

K8 Yasumoto, S. et al.: The combination restoration using glass-ionomer cement and composite resin. Evolution of glass-ionomer cements as a combination restorative material with composite resin, J.J. Conserv. Dent. 29(3): 856–865, 1986. (Japanese)

K9 Fujita, T.: Influence of microparticle filled resin restoration for pulp. Pulp protection effect of Dentin Adhesive Lining Material, J. Tokyo Dent. Coll. Soci. 86: 587–625, 1986. (Japanese)

K10 Herrin, H.K.: Use of a posterior composite resin to restore teeth and support enamel. Report of case, J.A.D.A. 112(Jun): 845–846, 1986.

K11 Hino H., and Onose, H.: Experimental of Adhesive force, for Composite resin and Glass-Ionomer Cement, J.J. Conserv. Dent. 30(2): 789–790, 1987. (Japanese)

K12 Yanagawa, T., and Kobayashi, Y.: Study on glass-ionomer cement as lining material. Part 1. Change of PH, J.J. Conserv. Dent. 30(2): 766–767, 1987. (Japanese)

K13 Narikawa, K.: Glass-ionomer cement as especially base material, J.J. Conserv. Dent. 30(7): 1987. (Japanese)

K14 Hino, H. et al.: Study on adhesive property for composite resin and glass-ionomer cement. Influence of composite resins polymerization for adhesive force, J.J. Conserv. Dent. 30: 89, 1987. (Japanese)

K15 Takamori, Y., and Ishikawa, T.: Protection of tooth substance for composite resin restoration, Quintessence 6: 37–52, 1987. (Japanese)

K16 Narikawa, K.: Lining (3) cement base, Dent. Diamond 12(9): 50–53, 1987. (Japanese)

K17 Causton, B. et al.: Bonding class II composite to etched glass ionomer cement, Br. Dent. J. 163(10): 321–324, 1987.

K18 Staehle, H.J.: Experimentelle untersuchungen über das löslichkeitsverhalten verschiedener unterfüllungsmaterialien, Dtsch. Zahnarztl. Z. 42(7): 633–638, 1987.

K19 Andreaus, S.B.: Liquid versus gel enchants on glass ionomers, Their effects on surface morphology and shear bond strengths to composite resins, J.A.D.A. 114(2): 157–158, 1987.

K20 Hinoura, K. et al.: Tensile bond strength between glass ionomer cements and composite resins, J.A.D.A. 114(2): 167–172, 1987.

K21 Crim, G.A., and Shay, J.S.: Microleakage pattern of a resin-veneered glass-ionomer cavity liner, J. Prosthet. Dent. 58(3): 273–276, 1987.

K22 Simokoube, H.: Adhesion of composite resin for base of glass-ionomer cement, J. Tokyo Dent. Ass. 6(4): 263–268, 1988. (Japanese)

K23 Bertolotti, R.L.: Removal of "black-line" margins and improving esthetics of porcelain-fused-to-metal crowns, Quintessence Int. 18(9): 645–647, 1987.

K24 Miyazaki, N.: Study on lining materials for composite resin restoration, J.J. Conserv. Dent. 31(3): 716–735, 1988. (Japanese)

K25 Hino, H., and Onose, H.: Study on sandwich technique, J. Dent. Med. 28(4): 429–435, 1988. (Japanese)

K26 Feilzer, A.J. et al.: Curing contraction of composites and glass-ionomer cements, J. Prosthet. Dent. 297–300, 1988.

K27 Smith, G.E.: Surface deterioration of glass-ionomer cement during acid etching. An SEM evaluation, Oper. Dent. 13: 3–7, 1988.

K28 Garcia-Godoy, F., and Malone, W,F.P.: Microleakage of posterior composite resins using glass ionomer cement bases, Quintessence Int. 19(1): 13–17, 1988.

K29 Wilson, H.J.: Resin-based restoratives, Br. Dent. J. 164(10): 326–330, 1988.

K30 Shortall, A.C., and Wilson, H.J.: New materials, bonding treatments and changes in restorative practice, Br. Dent. J. 164(12): 396–400, 1988.

L. Application for Fissure Sealant

L1 Takeuchi, M. et al.: Sealing of the pit and fissure with resin adhesive, I. II. Bull, Tokyo Dent. Coll. 7: 50–71, 1966.

L2 Cueto, E.I., and Buonocore, M.G.: Sealing of pits and fissures with an adhesive resin, its use in caries prevention, J.A.D.A. 75: 121–128, 1967.

L3 Buonocore, M.G.: Adhesive sealing of pits and fissures for caries prevention with ultraviolet light, J.A.D.A. 80: 324–328, 1970.

L4 McCune, R.J. *et al*.: Pit and fissure sealants, one year results from a study in kalispell. Montara, J.A.D.A. 87: 1177–1180, 1973.

L5 McLean, J.W., and Wilson, A.D.: Fissure sealing and filling with an adhesive glass-ionomer cement, Br. Dent. J. 136(2): 269–276, 1974.

L6 Masuhara, E., and Oomori, I.: Adhesion and anti-caries effect of MMA—TBB resin enamite, Quintessence Int. (4·5): 1–17, 1976.

L7 Williams, B., and Winter, G.B.: Fissure sealants, A 2-year clinical trial, Br. Dent. J. 141(1): 15–18, 1976.

L8 Kawakami, S.: The studies of pit and fissure sealant (2) On relation between demineralization and histological structure in the enamel surface of fissures, J.J. Conserv. Dent. 21: 565–580, 1978. (Japanese)

L9 Newbrun, E.: Cariology, 1978, The Williams & Wilkins Co..

L10 Williams, B. *et al*.: Fissure sealants, Br. Dent. J. 145(12): 359–364, 1978.

L11 Charbeneau, G.T., and Dennison, J.B.: Clinical success and potential failure after single application of a pit and fissure sealant. A four-year report, J.A.D.A. 98: 559–564, 1979.

L12 Williams, B., and Winter, G.B.: Fissure sealant—further results at 4 years, Br. Dent. J. 150(7): 183–187, 1981.

L13 Kawakami, S. *et al*.: Clinical records of glass-ionomer cement for fissure sealants, J. Hokkaido Dent. Ass. 37: 159–165, 1984. (Japanese)

L14 Kawakami, S. *et al*.: Signification of glass-ionomer cement for fissure sealants, Dent. Outlook 64(4): 749–758, 1984. (Japanese)

L15 Nishino, M.: Caries character of eruptions period of the permanent teeth, Dent. Outlook special issue. 95–103, 1984. (Japanese)

L16 Merz-Fairhurst, E.J. *et al*.: A comparative clinical study of two pit and fissure sealants. 7 year results in Augusta GA, J.A.D.A. 109: 252–255, 1984.

L17 Ripa, L.W.: The current status of pit and fissure sealants, A review, J. Canad. Dent. Assoc. 5: 367–380, 1985.

L18 Nakagawa, T. *et al*.: Influence of temperature change for glass-ionomer cement as fissure sealant and abrasion resistance, J.J. Conserv. Dent. 28(3): 1085, 1985. (Japanese)

L19 Hirota, K. *et al*.: Glass-ionomer cement for prophylactic plug in, J. Dent. Med. 24(1): 123, 1986. (Japanese)

L20 Yoshimura, M. *et al*.: The penetration of glass-ionomer cement sealant into pits and fissures, J.J. Conserv. Dent. 30(2): 527–534, 1987. (Japanese)

L21 Kawakami, S.: Q and A GC circle, 48, 33, 1986. (Japanese)

L22 Komatsu, H.: Glass-ionomer cement as fissure sealant, J.J. Conserv. Dent. 30: (Spring issue), 6, 1987. (Japanese)

L23 Yoshimura, M. *et al*.: Portative power and caries incidence rate for a year passaged glass-ionomer cement at the health center, J.J. Conserv. Dent. 30: (Spring issue), 93, 1987. (Japanese)

L24 Boksman, L. *et al*.: Clinical evaluation of a glass ionomer cement as a fissure sealant, Quintessence Int. 18(10): 707–709, 1987.

L25 McKenna, E.F., and Grundy, G.E.: Glass ionomer cement fissure sealants applied by operative dental auxiliaries retention rate after one year, Aust. Dent. J. 32(3): 200–203, 1987.

L26 Moriyasu, K., and Ohmori, I.: The latest one's way of thinking for prognosis of fissure sealant, J. Dent. Med. 27(6): 835–841, 1988. (Japanese)

L27 Miyakoshi, S. *et al*.: Relativity of fissure invasion and viscosity for fissure sealant glass-ionomer cement, J.J. Dent. Mater. Dev. 7: (Autumn issue), 1988. (Japanese)

L28 Komatsu, H. *et al*.: Enamel fluoride uptake from glass-ionomer cement, Designed for use as a fissure sealant. J.J. Conserv. Dent. 32: 688–695, 1989. (Japanese)

M. Metal Powder Combined Glass Ionomer

M1 Simmons, J.: The miracle mixture glass ionomer and alloy powder, Texas Dent. J. Oct. 6–12, 1983.

M2 McLean, J.W., and Gasser, O.: Glass-cermet cements, Quintessence Int. 5: 333–343, 1985.

M3 Croll, T.P., and Phillips, R.W.: Glass ionomer-silver cermet restorations for primary teeth, Quintessence Int. 17(10): 607–615, 1986.

M4 Mallakh, B. *et al*.: Does metal incorporation improve glass-ionomer properties? J. Dent. Res. 66(113): ABST50, 1987.

M5 Taleghani, M., and Morgan, R.W.: Reconstructive materials for endodontically treated teeth, J. Prosthet. Dent. 57(4): 446–449, 1987.

M6 Taleghani, M., and Leinfelder, K.F.: Evaluation of a new glass ionomer cement with silver as a core buildup under a cast restoration, Quintessence Int. 19(1): 19–24, 1988.

M7 Berg, J.H. *et al.*: Glass ionomer-silver restorations. A demineralization-remineralization, Quintessence Int. 19(9): 639–641, 1988.

M8 Croll, T.P.: Glass ionomer-silver cermet class II Tunnel-restorations for primary molars, J. Dent. Child. 55(3): 177–183, 1988.

M9 Tjan, A.H.L., and Morgan, D.L.: Metal-reinforced glass ionomers. Their flexural and bond strengths to tooth substrates, J. Prosthet. Dent. 59(2): 137–141, 1988.

M10 Sarkar, N.K. *et al.*: Silver release from metal-reinforced glass ionomers, Dent. Mater. 4: 103–104, 1988.

M11 Reich, E. *et al.*: Haftfestigkeit von materialien zum aufbau vitaler zaehne, Dtsch. Zahnarztl. Z. 43(8): 847–850, 1988.

M12 Hickel, R. *et al.*: Nachuntersuchung von füellungen mit cermet-zement (Ketac-Silver), Dtsch. Zahnarztl. Z. 43(8): 851–853, 1988.

M13 Hickel, R.: Erste klinische ergebnisse von retrograden wurzelfüllungen mit cermet-zement, Dtsch. Zahnarztl. Z. 43(9): 963–965, 1988.

M14 Baraban, D.J.: The restoration of endodontically treated teeth. An update, J. Prosthet. Dent. 59(5): 553–559, 1988.

M15 Stratmann, R.G. *et al.*: Class II glass ionomer-silver restorations in primary molars, Quintessence Int. 20(1): 43–47, 1989.

N. Etching of Smear Layer

N1 Duke, E.S. *et al.*: Effects of various agents in cleaning cut dentine, J. Oral Rehabil. 12: 295–302, 1985.

N2 Berry III, E.A. *et al.*: Dentin surface treatments for the removal of the smear layer, J.A.D.A. 115(1): 65–67, 1987.

N3 Croll, T.P.: Repair of severe crown fracture with glass ionomer and composite resin bonding, Quintessence Int. 19(9): 649–653, 1988.

N4 Hunter, J.K. *et al.*: The repair of a lateral resorptive root defect with a glass ionomer cement. A case report, Quintessence Int. 17(9): 523–532, 1986.

N5 McLean, J.W.: A new method of bonding dental cements and porcelain to metal, Oper. Dent. 2: 130-, 1977.

N6 Vitsentzos, S.I.: Study of the retention of pins, J. Prosthet. Dent. 60(4): 447–451, 1988.

O. Etc.

O1 McLean, J.W.: The future of restorative materials, J. Prosthet. Dent. 42, 154–158, 1979.

O2 Irie, M.: Study on adhesive properties for Glass-Ionomer Cement, J.J. Res. Sci. Dent. Mater. Appli. 38(2): 250–289, 1981. (Japanese)

O3 Croll, T.P.: Repair of severe crown fracture with glass ionomer and composite resin bonding, Quintessence Int. 19(9): 649–653, 1988.